Caring for Persons with AIDS and Cancer

Ethical Reflections on Palliative Care for the Terminally Ill

John F. Tuohey, PhD

Visiting Assistant Professor of Moral Theology
Department of Religion & Religious Education
The Catholic University of America

The Catholic Health Association of the United States
St. Louis, MO

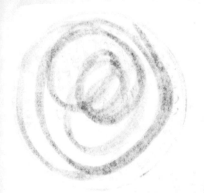

Library of Congress Cataloging-in-Publication Data

Tuohey, John F.
  Caring for persons with AIDS and cancer.

  Includes bibliographies and index.
    1. AIDS (Disease)—Patients—Palliative treatment—
Moral and ethical aspects.   2. Cancer—Patients—
Palliative treatment—Moral and ethical aspects.
3. Terminal care—Moral and ethical aspects.   I. Title.
[DNLM: 1. Acquired Immunodeficiency Syndrome.
2. Attitude to Death.   3. Ethics, Medical.   4. Neoplasms.
5. Palliative Treatment.   6. Terminal Care.
WB 310 T927c]
RC607.A26T86   1988   174'.24   88-11806
ISBN 0-87125-150-7   Rev.

Copyright 1988
by
The Catholic Health Association of the United States
4455 Woodson Road
St. Louis, MO 63134-0889

Printed in the United States of America.

Table of Contents

THE PERSON
Personality and Character
Past and Future
Culture
Roles
Relationships
Political Aspect
Doer of Things
Body
Secret Life
Transcendence
Integration

The "person" is primary in all things.

The moral imperative is to relieve suffering and to facilitate the living person in achieving well-being.

Physical death is not an absolute evil; physical life is not an absolute value.

The will of the patient is fundamental for well-being.

The patient/family is the unit of care.

Artificial procedures for maintaining adequate levels of nourishment and hydration are life-prolonging therapies that, as with other life-prolonging therapies, may be withheld or withdrawn when they offer the person no benefit with respect to well-being in physical living or dying.

The use of narcotics for the control of severe chronic pain is appropriate medical therapy.

Reconciliation with death is possible.

Persons die in their own time.

Palliative care is an appropriate modality of care for the terminally ill.

CONCLUSION

List of
Figures and Tables

LIST OF FIGURES

LIST OF TABLES

Acknowledgements

When I began research for this work, originally as a doctoral dissertation, I began with the decision to ground myself in the medical reality with which I was dealing. I am especially grateful to the people of the Palliative Care Unit of Western Massachusetts Hospital, Westfield, MA, for assisting me in doing this. Working with and among them, I gained many of the medical and personal insights that inform this work.

I wish also to acknowledge the contribution of Paul *Schotsmans, Professor of Ethics in the Faculty of Medicine of the University of Louvain, Belgium, who directed the doctoral dissertation that became the foundation of this present work. I am indebted to Anne Costa, whose assistance in editing the original dissertation helped lay the groundwork necessary for its expansion. I am also grateful to my students at the University of Massachusetts, Amherst, MA, and at The Catholic University of America, Washington, DC, for their questions and comments that helped me to refine my thoughts and presentation.

Finally, I wish to acknowledge the encouragement of colleagues and friends, and the support and understanding of my family. It is with deep gratitude that I acknowledge them here.

Introduction

Nearly 25,000 people have died in the United States with acquired immune deficiency syndrome (AIDS). There are approximately 400 new cases of AIDS diagnosed each month. Each year, approximately 450,000 people die in the United States with cancer. That means that over 1,000 people will die with cancer every day. These are sobering facts that raise critical questions: How shall we care for people who cannot be cured? What is appropriate care for the terminally ill?

The need for better answers to these questions is evident by the confusion often found within the medical field in its care for the dying. Often, the dying are treated as if they are going to get better and go home, when actually they are not going to get better and, if they do go home, it will be to die there. At other times, the person is emotionally or even physically abandoned because it is thought that nothing more can be done. People who are dying often find themselves in the rooms farthest from the nurses' station, have to wait longer for a response to a call for assistance, and often receive no attention at all near the end of a shift lest the discovery of their death interrupt the daily schedule. It is sometimes forgotten that people who are dying are still living.

The purpose of this book is to propose an ethical framework for palliative care as an answer to the question of appropriate care for the terminally ill. Some aspects of ethical reasoning found in acute and chronic care may be inappropriate for the care of the dying. The needs of the person are different, and the methods of care in one modality do not always easily adapt to another. Past efforts to appeal to acute and chronic care reasoning for those who cannot be cured have led to instances of people being subject to invasive and costly procedures, as well as being sustained on life-support systems that offer no benefit. One study also revealed the frequency of the simultaneous, and rather contradictory, initiation of one life-sustaining procedure as another is removed.[1]

To begin to answer the question of care, it is first necessary to know the purpose of care. For that, it is mandatory to understand what it means to be a patient. Ramsey has written that healthcare professionals must always keep in mind that the patient is a person.[2] I fully agree. Still, that is not enough. Not only is the patient a person, but this person is also a patient. That is, the personhood of the individual is somehow affected or threatened with the onset of some illness or trauma. Unless there is a clear understanding of what it means to be a patient, it will be impossible to understand the goals of medicine in regard to the person. This is the purpose of the first two chapters of this book: to describe what it means to be a patient; that is, to show how personhood is threatened by disease and illness so that the goals of medicine may be clearly defined and pursued.

The person who is dying is a particular kind of patient. He or she is a patient who is presented with threats to personal integrity by the disease that are not going to pass and who faces a whole other set of threats. Those are the threats associated with death. These, too, need to be understood. Without a clear understanding of what it means to be dying and how people cope with that reality, it will be impossible to know the needs of the dying person. If there is no accurate conception of the person's needs, there will be no opportunity to offer appropriate care.

With this as a foundation, I will present an illustration of palliative care as it is practiced in the United States. Here I will make specific reference to the Palliative Care Unit at Western Massachusetts Hospital in Westfield; without the assistance of the healthcare professionals at this institution, this book could never have been written. My purpose in this presentation is simply to describe what already happens in care. Palliative care is different from acute and chronic care. These modalities of care are not exclusive, yet they do have different methods and goals. The methods of one may be inappropriate for the achievement of the goals of another. Once it is understood what it means to be a dying patient, it should be clear that appropriate care will be that care seeking to respond to the needs of that person. Life-sustaining care may not speak to the needs of the person who is dying.

Finally, this book will offer an ethical reflection on the practice of palliative care. This reflection will not be based on preconceived ethical principles, although those principles will be of great importance. Also, this reflection will not be based on a comparison of palliative care with the goals and methods of acute and chronic care, even though a comparison is helpful. Instead, this reflection will attempt to discover how well palliative care, as it is currently practiced, meets the goals of medicine.

How shall we care for the many thousands of people in our society for whom traditional medicine will not work? This book is meant not so much to offer an answer as to give an ethical reflection on the answer proposed by palliative care and hospice. The care is there. What I hope to do is demonstrate that what is sometimes called an innovation in care—a type of care outside the mainstream of medicine, a "there is nothing more we can do" kind of care, or a legitimization of passive euthanasia—is, in fact, nothing of the sort. Palliative care is simply one of three modes of care that seek to respond to the needs of the person who has, for whatever reason, become a patient. Acute care is unique because it assists the person in moving toward a full recovery, chronic care because it allows the person to live meaningfully with whatever limitations may result from the illness or trauma, and palliative care because it allows the person to live out one's own death. By recalling to mind the goals of medicine, it is possible to see that what palliative care and hospice offer is not new but simply reflects a rediscovery and, perhaps, a greater appreciation and application of what has always been appropriate care: helping the person to live well.

NOTES

1. Kenneth Micetich, Patricia Steinecker, and David Thomasma, "Are Intravenous Fluids Morally Required for a Dying Patient?" *Archives of Internal Medicine* 143, 1983, pp. 975-978. This study revealed that almost all the physicians interviewed would initiate intravenous therapy for a patient facing imminent death or in an irreversible coma, yet they would be willing to remove a respirator.
2. Paul Ramsey, *The Patient as Person: Explorations in Medical Ethics,* Yale University Press, New Haven, 1970.

1 / *The Person and Well-Being*

Whenever a person is ill or suffers some trauma, the person as a whole is affected. Describing that effect on the person, we say that the person becomes a patient. That is, the person presents him/herself as one who stands in some medical need. The purpose of this first chapter is to describe who this person is and what it means to be a patient.

In doing this, it will also be necessary to study the meaning of health and sickness. This will make it possible to articulate the goals of healthcare. Without an understanding of the fundamental distinction between health and sickness and a clear understanding of the goals of medicine, it will not be possible to reflect on the ethical appropriateness of any mode of care.

Finally, the chapter will close with a look at two paradigms for care. The first will reflect a more traditional approach, understanding health as having to do with the physical abilities of the person. The second, following from the discussion concerning personhood and the goals of medicine, will offer a more holistic approach to what will be described as personal well-being.

THE PERSON

The person who is the object of concern in medicine and moral thought is not an object at all. Rather, the person is a subject, a subject who happens to be in need. As a subject, the person can never be reduced to any of his/her needs. Personal integrity and dignity always transcend needs.

One of the temptations easily fallen into in the medical field is to see the person as a collection of tissues, organs, and systems. When this happens, the task of the medical profession becomes that of maintenance: keep tissues, organs, and systems operating. When they fail to do so on their own, they are to be given some chemical or mechanical assistance. When and if that also fails, they are to be replaced. Should even that fail, there is

1

nothing more that can be done, and the situation is regarded as being hopeless.

If the person were, in fact, merely a collection of biological entities, then these certainly would be the goals, although simplistically stated, of medicine. Such, however, is not the case. The person is not merely a collection of biological realities. As Reidy points out:

> *It is wise to select various aspects of the human being which we can understand fully, when by so doing we can apply in a helpful way the knowledge we gain. But equally, it is foolish to pretend that when we have successfully isolated the working of the tissue, or the patterns of the mind, that we are then in possession of a total understanding of man.*[1]

One of the points Ramsey helps to illuminate, by bringing together both the Roman Catholic and the other-Christian traditions, is that the focus on one set of realities can never take precedence over the other.[2] Although other-Christian traditions are free from a strictly "physical benefits" theory with regard to the person and thus are able to transcend the merely physical, the Roman Catholic tradition, precisely because of its emphasis on physical benefits, does safeguard the need for an appropriate concern for embodied existence and the integrity of the flesh. In short, the person is not body *and* spirit, but a totality of being. As Häring express it:

> *Traditionally, the Christian doctrine of man's nature states that man is a composite of body and spirit, but one cannot construe addivity. It would be inaccurate to say that man* has *a body. Man is an embodied spirit; he* is *a live body.*[3]

The person, presenting him/herself as a patient, does so as a whole being. This wholeness is, of course, a subject. For all the information we may have about a certain individual or the illness, there is never an object of care, but always a subject participating in care.

Who then is this total subject in healthcare? There have been many attempts in various disciplines to articulate the characteristics that make up the whole person.[4] As a framework on which to build my own insights, I will use those characteristics outlined by Cassel.[5] It is appropriate that any work in bioethics begin with the medical reality, drawing insights from the medical profession. Cassel's multidimensional presentation of the person is particularly well suited for this.

Personality and Character

Cassel begins by describing the person as a being having personality and character. These appear and begin to develop in the first few weeks of life and remain with the person for extended periods during, and possibly all, the person's life. Personality exerts a great deal of influence on the way the person copes with an illness or some trauma in life. This observation is supported by such research as done by Simonton et al.[6] Differences in personality and character development can perhaps account for the situation that sometimes appears when two people have the same prognosis, yet one will live whereas the other dies. Says Cassel:

Some people do in fact have stronger characters and bear adversity better. Some are good and kind under the stress of terminal illness, whereas others become mean and offensive when even mildly ill.[7]

Past and Future

Persons have a past—a history, a biography. People who become ill do so with a memory of past health and illness. This history accompanies them and influences their thoughts and actions. Cassel states further that memory exists not only in the mind, but also "in the nostrils and the hands. . . . A fragrance drifts by, and a memory is evoked. My feet have not forgotten how to roller-skate."[8] Memory of one's history stimulates anxiety in some and confidence in others:

Even if it is fatal, the disease may not produce the destruction of the person, but rather, reaffirm his or her indomitability.[9]

Just as persons have a past, so too do they enjoy a future. A future consists of the plans and aspirations one holds. A change in one's health will have a profound effect on this future by introducing physical, emotional, or financial limitations that can make future prospects bleak or impossible. The future also contains expectations for others and one's participation in that. Often, one's future depends to a greater or lesser degree on another's presence and support. To the extent this is true, futures merge, as when a child's athletic career becomes one with a parent who has spent hours developing skills and attending games. When a person becomes ill, he/she may see not only one's own future endangered, but the future of others as well. In the same way, one may see his/her future begin to fade in the illness of another on whom he/she has come to depend. This double grief can have a profound impact on life.

Culture

Persons exist within a cultural setting. The powerful influence that culture can have on one's view of illness and death should not be underestimated. Western culture, for example, often has difficulty expressing concern for those with no obvious symptoms. In one instance, a young man's religious superior asked him to please begin to use a crutch, since this would make it easier to believe that the young man truly was experiencing pain in his healthy-looking left leg. As will be described in Chapter Three, culture can also influence how people grieve. A brief example that illustrates this point involves two cultures that did not mix. A Filipino woman's husband of 12 years died in a drowning accident. At the graveside service, the widow threw herself onto her husband's coffin in grief. Although in the Philippines this is certainly acceptable behavior, such action here in the United States led her American husband's family to believe that she was insane with grief. Such unfair accusations based on cultural expectations only made the widow's grieving all the more difficult.

Roles

All people have certain roles in society and in their more immediate social area. Persons often identify themselves in their roles and, by so doing, take on certain norms that define and clarify their own identity. Cassel goes on to state that, by middle age, roles may be so firmly set that disease can lead to the virtual destruction of a person by making the performance of those roles impossible. Whatever the role, when someone cannot perform his/her duties, the person is diminished.

Relationships

Persons exist in relationships; they cannot exist alone. "Take away others, remove sight or hearing, and the person is diminished."[10] This can happen physically through some injury or emotionally through some change in the status of relationships. Disease can precipitate changes in either instance, the physical being the more obviously affected. Disease or infection can cause scar tissue that is perceived as repulsive, inhibit some faculty, or even necessitate the removal of some organ or limb that may be instrumental in promoting relationships.

Relationships are the context within which our emotions find their expression; take away this context and our emotional selves are impoverished. Loss of some physical function, such as sexual performance, or a dramatic change in one's appearance can influence a breakdown in relationships. This can result from the withdrawal of the patient from others or the avoidance of the patient by others. Fear of contagion also plays a role in relationships. This fear on the part of others often keeps people away. The result is isolation.

Political Aspect

Cassel uses political language to indicate that all persons are equal under law, with rights and obligations and the ability to seek recourse for injury. Illness affects these rights, obligations, and privileges. As will be shown, people with acquired immune deficiency syndrome (AIDS) or cancer are often denied employment or must accept employment without medical benefits. This can bring about in the patient a sense of powerlessness and lack of appreciation.

Doer of Things

Illness or trauma can infringe on the person's ability to perform. This, in turn, can have a profound effect on one's perception of oneself and on how the person is perceived by others. Underlying this is an understanding of the self as a doer. Persons do things and perform acts. The person also understands how to make things happen. This somewhat unconscious awareness is affected in illness. In many instances, people cannot explain why they feel the way they do, nor can they understand why they can no longer do the things they used to do or why they now perform certain acts:

> *People can behave in ways that seem inexplicable and strange even to themselves, and the sense of powerlessness that the person may feel in the presence of such behavior can be a source of great distress.* [11]

One young gentleman described himself as having a type of inferiority complex because of his illness. This caused him to question the motivation of those who were kind to him while he was ill.

Body

As mentioned in the discussion of the patient as a subject, each person is an "embodied spirit." [12] It is in and through the body that the spiritedness of the person projects an image to oneself and to others. This is sometimes referred to as *body image*. [13] Persons trust their bodies to perform in certain ways and to be presented favorably to others. In illness, one's body can be altered, along with others' image or perception of the person. Some people may assume that their acceptance is based on appearance and will work for changes in the body that facilitate this; body building or diet control, for example, may be desirable activities. On the other hand, any change that will detract from one's appearance, such as the excessive weight loss that often accompanies AIDS and cancer, is undesirable.

Body image is tied closely to one's self-concept.[14] People tend to think highly of themselves when they look good and perform well; as appearance is distorted, self-esteem may be lowered.

This understanding of the self as a body can be taken further. All bodies are limited and function within the limits of space and time. This is part of the human condition. This can be seen as a limiting and negative aspect of our existence or as a positive description of humanity. Regardless of the outlook, disease or trauma can change that perception. If people see themselves as being limited by the body, then any further restriction in performance will only aggravate that vision. If one has the more optimistic outlook of seeing natural, physical limitedness as an opportunity and challenge, then to see these change is to see opportunities fade; challenges can become obstacles that may appear, and in fact may be, insurmountable.

Secret Life

Unknown to others is that part of one's life that is secret. All persons have some aspect of privacy or secrecy in life. This secret life may exist in reality or only in the imagination. In either case, it is nevertheless perceived as being real. At times, it is this secret life that keeps the rest of one's public life manageable or tolerable. Illness may introduce an obstacle to living out this secret as the patient loses privacy. Also, a secret person may have no legitimate place at the sickbed. The loss of this person "can be a source of great distress and intensely private pain."[15]

A person's secret life may be particularly affected in cases of AIDS. In circumstances where AIDS is identified with homosexuality, there is often a tendency to judge people as unworthy of care because of the perceived inappropriateness of their behavior. In such cases, the illness may expose one's secret life, raising difficulties with family or friends, employment, and so forth. Even in cases where the person with AIDS is not involved in any prejudged behavior, the "secret" of having AIDS or testing positive for the virus, when it is known, can lead to a complete ruin of one's life. In this instance, the disease may introduce the need for a secret life that the person does not want and is not prepared to live.

Transcendence

Cassel also speaks of the person's transcendent nature, that quality of being greater and more lasting than an individual life, giving the person a timeless dimension. It is when the person is reduced to any one aspect of personhood that there is the danger of losing sight of this human transcendence. If this aspect of the person is ignored or forgotten, his/her ability to rise above the current distress, the ability to resort to one's inner resources, can be limited.

As will be seen later, disease itself is rooted in the person, as is one's ability to recover from, or at least cope with, that illness. Unless the spirit is free to transcend the current crisis, the person will not be able to "own" that illness, and his/her ability to recover may be compromised. In this respect, the medical profession itself must be transcendent. It must be able to transcend the physical body that comes before it and see the person who is ill.

Integration

A characteristic that I would add to Cassel's list is the ability to integrate or synthesize. It is one thing to say that the person consists of the characteristics just listed, but these also must be somehow brought together into a coherent and whole being. This is the ability to integrate. Cassel, as well as many others, does not refer to this. As will be seen, however, it is an important characteristic that plays a central role in determining the appropriateness or inappropriateness of care with respect to the ill, especially the terminally ill, person.

Without this ability to integrate, the person can never be a whole, remaining instead a collection of independent characteristics. Lifton and Olson make the point that to be human is to experience a quest for integrity, movement, and connection.[16] Munley calls this "a movement toward synthesis."[17] This quest or movement involves a reflection on life experiences, assessing successes and failures, and assigning meaning to the entire experience of life.

I am speaking here of the ability to pull things together into a coherent and meaningful whole, making sense of reality so that it can be lived. Illness or some trauma can have a profound effect on this ability to integrate. For example, the person integrates the body with a personality and achieves a certain balance of activity in life style. When the person's body is challenged, this person's wholeness or integrity will be threatened. That is, not only is their body threatened, but personhood is threatened as well. This same person will have to begin again to seek a new integration,

7

bringing together new information concerning the body. This could involve finding a meaningful life style with an artificial limb or merely coping with being laid up in bed for a few weeks.

Integration involves all characteristics of the person, each working in and through the other characteristics to keep the person in balance and in control of one's destiny. Roberts illustrates this psychological process by using a physical parallel:

> *When one body system loses equilibrium, all other systems also become involved. Normally the individual mobilizes patterns of defense to re-establish or maintain equilibrium. An individual who trips over a throw rug, for example, mobilizes his entire body toward maintaining or restoring equilibrium to keep him from falling. If he succeeds, he will simply stumble, but if he fails, the individual will try to get himself in a state of readiness to be protected from injury as he falls.[18]*

I will refer to this process as the *pursuit of the human task;* that is, the effort to integrate all that a person is with the self and the world in order to place or discover some order and meaning in life. The purpose of life is to do just that: to place or discover the meaning of life. To do this is to pursue the human task.

Life and its events do not necessarily contain an inherent meaning. Although it is convenient to explain what happens in life in this way, not every event that happens does so for any particular reason. Likewise, illness does not necessarily mean anything. It just is. Persons place or discover meaning in what occurs. In this sense, they make life meaningful by making life full of meaning.

For example, after a cardiac arrest, I may learn to slow down and enjoy some of life's other beauties besides my work. That does not mean, however, that I had a heart attack to learn to slow down. Whatever meaning is there I have discovered in reflecting on the events of my life and seeing how they all seem to unfold in a unified whole. Or, I may have placed this meaning in my life by interpreting that event in the light of some religious or philosophical framework I have freely chosen as the ground of my understanding.

The task of each human person, the human task, is to place or discover some meaning in life's events. This may be health, illness, or even death. When this is done, when I have integrated all that I am with my whole self and the world around me, life makes sense. My health, my illness, and even my dying have meaning. When life's events have meaning, it is possible to live them out—even the most difficult and painful ones.

I use the expression "place or discover" here because people do both. At times, we are quite original in how we understand our lives, drawing on the insights of others in ways that are new and often surprising. In that sense, we place meaning in our life. At other times, perhaps more often, we see a hint of meaning in the unfolding of the event or we take as our own some religious or philosophical insights that others have offered from their own pursuit. In this case, it might be said that we are placing meaning in our lives, taking as our own what another has found helpful.

In either case, whether placing, discovering, or combining the two, the person is seeking to integrate his/herself with reality to make some sense out of it. When this cannot be done, when the human task is obstructed, there is the experience of meaninglessness and perhaps despair. When this can be done, when the human task of placing or discovering order and meaning in life can be pursued, then life has meaning. It is only when life has meaning that it becomes possible to live it out. As one person with AIDS stated, "AIDS was the best thing that ever happened to me. It forced me to get my life together."

It is apparent then that any threat to any characteristic of the person will be a threat to the integrity or wholeness of the entire person and a disruption of the human task. The greater the threat or the perception of that threat, the greater is the effect on personal integrity and the more meaningless the situation may appear.

Disease and the possibility of death are examples of just such threats. They require an appropriate response. As will be seen in greater detail, it is that response which allows the person enough control within his/her life situation to facilitate the pursuit of the human task that is most appropriate.

It is essential that the integratedness of the many different characteristics of the person be understood before any ethical statement can be made concerning medical care. If this is forgotten, there is a danger of isolating the person from him/herself by making decisions for that person that, although they may specifically address the disease, may not help the person to exercise some control within the situation. The person may thus be denied the opportunity to give meaning to life in general and to the illness or dying in particular.

HEALTH AND SICKNESS

Health

Saying that the person's integrity is threatened by sickness and that the person seeks health, raises the two questions: What is health? and What is

9

meant by sickness? Indeed, the distinction between health and sickness provides the first and most fundamental ethical insight into medical care. If there is no proper perception of health and sickness, then the goal of medicine will be obscured.

The definition proposed here will not be a medical definition as such. In view of the holistic approach I have taken, a definition rooted in any exact science would be inadequate. Instead, I will propose a more anthropological definition.

Tillich's pastoral psychology offers a good starting point for understanding what is meant by health. He offers six characteristics of health:[19]

1. *Physical:* an adequate function of biological parts
2. *Chemical:* appropriate balance of chemical substances and processes
3. *Biological:* appropriate interaction of the self as an organism with its total environment, including rest, movement, food, and other functions
4. *Psychological:* appropriate balance between a secure sense of personal identity (finding oneself) and the ability to lose the self in love of others
5. *Social and historical:* to some extent, personal health depends on the health and sanity of society (as well as, I would add, genetic inheritance)
6. *Spiritual:* the awareness of and capacity for being grasped by the spirit, that source and meaning of life that transcends the person yet is not foreign to his/her innermost being

This multidimensional perspective of health is shared in other writings as well.[20] Health, therefore, is much more than most think; it is more than physical vitality and capabilities. Health also involves the part of the self that is not physical.

Health is multidimensional, having to do with a whole and integrated balance of personhood. Health also involves the person's integration with what is outside the self, such as the world, culture, and some ultimate reality. Any other definition of health is too narrow and encourages a reduction of the person to only one or a few characteristics. If health were merely physical, then no attention needs to be given to the psychological or spiritual dimension of the person, and no concern needs to be shown for another's past or secret life. With this as a foundation, I propose the following as a tentative working definition: health is a state of optimal functioning or well-being.

The key element in this definition is expressed in the word "optimal." Optimal does not refer to some predetermined, standard level of function, with one's personal health being determined in relation to that. Health involves optimal functioning in that it has to do with the best function possible within a given situation. As such, health involves an integration and balance that allows a person to function in life in the best manner that he/she is able.

This definition reflects the idea that a condition of health encompasses much more than the physical in its reference to the person. Further, this condition does not have to be perfect or even close to perfect. Instead, it must be "optimal," that is, the best for a particular time, person, and circumstance. These are important concepts because they move away from a narrow view that would be tied to a strictly physical approach in medical care, broadening this to include care for the whole person. If it is the goal of medicine to restore the person to health, this definition gives important insights into what ought to be done for a particular person in a particular situation to achieve it. It is not possible to bring a person to health by merely addressing one characteristic of the person. Healing in one dimension of the person will not necessarily bring healing to the other dimensions or to the whole.

This definition of health recalls the earlier statement describing the person as one who integrates or seeks to achieve a balance or equilibrium in life between all aspects of personhood. If the person is to become an integrated whole, then he/she must be able to exercise some control within the environment and circumstances in which the person is found. This would not be an absolute control, but rather a control within one's pursuit of the human task. In this sense, control may be defined as the ability to do what needs to be done in order to facilitate integration and wholeness. Health requires some control within one's life and environment, some control and active participation within the healing process in order to facilitate this integration. Medical care should not be done "to" or "for" a patient, but rather "with" the patient. Such a view allows for the health of the vulnerable, the weak, the handicapped, and the elderly person, thus preserving the dignity of the person and human condition in all phases of life and in each of life's situations. This includes death. The goal of the medical care profession is not necessarily to return the patient to a previous physical condition; sometimes this is not possible. Nor is it to merely keep the person alive, as if simply existing constituted a state of health; it does not. Living encompasses a broad range of life experiences of which death is a part. The meaning and value of life is misunderstood if there is only an interest in physical capabilities or in the number of years a person exists.

The goal of medical care is to facilitate the integration of personhood in the present condition whether that is a moment of birthing, vitality, weakness, or dying. Medicine assists the patient by healing and strengthening that person to live fully the human response to life. That response is not so much threatened by the limitations inherent in human living or by death as it is when the opportunity to place or discover meaning in life has been taken away.

If health is defined in the broad and seemingly more accurate sense as the optimal functioning of the person in his/her wholeness in a particular set of circumstances, then health involves a general sense of well-being that arises from the ability to exercise personhood in integrating oneself and one's environment. This is possible only when the person is able to exercise some control within the present state of affairs, whether happiness and physical health, the occurrence of some acute crisis, the need for some modification in one's life style, or getting on with the human task of dying. This concept is reflected in the goals of cancer rehabilitation at the Los Angeles County–University of Southern California Cancer Center, where it is stated that the quality of survival is found not in how long a person lives, but in how well that person lives within the constraints of the disease.[21]

Sickness

Health, as already defined, is a multidimensional concept. It follows that sickness, too, will be multidimensional. This can be illustrated by examining sickness from three perspectives: physiological, ontological, and psychosomatic.

Physiological Illness. In his works on the history of medicine, Oswei refers to the physiological concept of disease.[22] This concept explains disease as the result of a breakdown of the internal physical balance of the person caused by some excess or defect in the function of one or more organs. This internal dysfunction ultimately results in illness. For example, an abnormal liver function could lead to excessive amounts of bile in a person's body fluids, leading to a condition known as jaundice. In this approach, changes in one's life style and diet may be viewed as being more important than the use of medicines. Such a concept is not without some merit, as will be seen later in a discussion of the psychosomatic elements of illness.

Ontological Illness. Oswei also refers to the ontological concept of disease. By this, Oswei means that diseases exist as separate entities, such as devils, contagions, bacteria, neuroses, or psychoses, that can be named, classified, and dealt with. The person fights off these invaders with specific drugs for specific diseases.

McGill makes reference to this ontological approach when he describes public awareness of illness and suffering as being a form of violence that strikes people.[23] McGill notes that, in news reports, what is most often reported is not what people do, but what happens to them: a man does not die in a bank robbery, he *is* killed. Like violence, illness is described as being inflicted on someone:

> *Eighty years ago, you got sick because of some weakening or impediment in the power of life that* naturally *belonged to the body. Therefore, to be healed, you don't put power in, but make use of one's own natural vitality. Today we see illness as an invasion from some* outside *power into them.*[24]

This "from without" attitude toward illness is often reflected in medicine. If the resources of one's own body are not sufficient, then one "fights fire with fire." According to McGill, to the extent that people see themselves victimized by powers, they invent other powers to deal with them: machines, drugs, and so forth. "In other words, against the obscure and occult forces of disease they have recourse to obscure counter forces."[25]

The ontological approach is not unfamiliar to different religious traditions. In the Judeo-Christian tradition, health and sickness have sometimes been understood to be expressions of God's favor or judgment on a person. Although such an understanding is theologically inappropriate, it does continue to inform some people's attitudes in selective, and perhaps self-serving, instances. AIDS, for example, has been referred to by former Moral Majority Director Jerry Falwell as "a lethal judgment of God on America for endorsing this vulgar, perverted, and reprobate lifestyle."[26]

Another example, coming from a different religious tradition, is found in Hinduism. In Hindu thought, people's experiences of reality are described and explained through their relationships with the three forms of God: Brahma, creator of the universe; Vishnu, preserver of the universe, and Krishna, the destroyer of the universe.[27] The emphasis of evil befalling on one from without can be seen in the great popularity and numerous temples of Krishna. When asked why there was so much devotion to a destroyer, rather than to a creator or preserver, one Hindu replied that precisely because Krishna destroys, "it is better to stay on his good side."[28]

Psychosomatic Illness. Often the term *psychosomatic*[29] is taken to mean that someone's illness is "all in the head." The implication is that the disease does not really exist. This is inaccurate. Psychosomatic is used to indicate that an illness originated as a result of, or is aggravated by, an individual's psychological processes. The illness is no less real just because it does not have a solely physical origin. In fact, most illnesses can be said to be psychosomatic.

Studies in this area have been made with the use of what is known as biofeedback. Biofeedback refers to the ability to exercise influence over bodily functions previously thought to be uninfluenced by conscious efforts. Studies have shown that it is possible, for example, to control voluntarily one's heart rate, muscle tension, sweat gland activity, and skin temperature, as well as a wide range of other conditions previously thought to be influenced only by the central nervous system (CNS) and therefore strictly involuntary.[30]

Through similar studies, Elmer and Alyce Green of the Menninger Clinic have found that every change in a person's physiological state is accompanied by a corresponding change in the mental-emotional state, either consciously or unconsciously. Conversely, every change in one's mental-emotional state, conscious or unconscious, is accompanied by a corresponding change in the physiological state.[31]

Simonton et al. suggest that these data have helped to move the orientation of medicine away from the idea that the body is an object needing repairs and spare parts to an understanding that the mind and body are elements of an integrated system.[32] Such an observation supports the contention put forward here that the person is a whole, brought together by the person's ability to integrate the self with the self and the environment, and that health has to do with the degree of this integration. When this integration is lacking, for whatever reason, health is lessened. Restoring a person to health, therefore, has to do with more than focusing on the disease. Medical care must also take into consideration the whole person in order that his/her integrity can be restored. Integrity or wholeness needs to be restored, or a cure may not be attained, but merely the semblance of cure. The true reasons behind the illness may remain.

Moving from Sickness to Health

A synthesis of the preceding concepts illustrates that sickness is the result of a loss of balance within and between internal and outside influences. To the degree that internal harmony is preserved, health is maintained and outside influences will be unable to make an impact on the person. One's ability to maintain health, however, is not absolute. When the environment changes beyond a certain range, being in many respects relative to the individual, the person may no longer be able to maintain internal harmony and function at previous levels or even at all if the change is extreme. The amount of oxygen, variations in temperature, and the presence of certain levels of bacteria are a few examples of outside conditions that can fluctuate within or beyond the range in which the person can live. What is important to keep in mind, however, is that the influence exterior factors exert on the person's health is largely relative to the extent that this is made possible by the person's own internal harmony.

When sickness does affect a person, that person's integrity is threatened. This is clear from the understanding of illness as being the result of internal and external factors. Ashley addresses this integrity:

> ... *[integrity] indicates that in a perfect whole each part must be fully differentiated and developed. Furthermore, each part must be fitted into the whole and harmonized with it by correct interrelation and interactions with the other parts of the whole. Integrity is lacking when a part is suppressed or unduly inhibited in function or when, on the other hand, one part is hypertrophied to the injury of others.*[33]

The threat illness poses to this integrity can be seen in two ways. On the one hand, integrity or wholeness may be lacking, resulting in the loss of internal harmony that allowed for illness in the first place. In this case, the real threat to the person derives from some internal or personal difficulty that has disrupted integrity, for example, stress over one's career. On the other hand, when the environment contains conditions that exceed the body's limited ability to maintain internal harmony, the threat to the person's integrity is posed directly by the disease itself as it begins to disrupt one's internal harmony.

Whether one's wholeness is disrupted by the disease or the disease results from a lack of wholeness on the part of the person, the result is the same: the person's integrity is disrupted. To the extent that this disrupts the person's pursuit of the human task, life will appear to be meaningless.

PARADIGM OF WELL-BEING

In discussions of health and sickness, the person may be traditionally viewed as being on a linear continuum, moving back and forth between the two extremes. Such a paradigm might be presented visually as shown in Fig. 1.1.

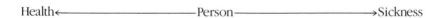

Health ←————————————Person————————————→ Sickness

Fig. 1.1 Paradigm of Health

Insofar as the person matches certain expectations of health, such as heart rate, blood pressure, and cholesterol count, the person might be said

15

to move closer to the health end of the spectrum and might be described as being more or less healthy depending on how close he/she is to that end. As fewer and fewer of these characteristics can be ascribed to the person, he/she is said to move toward the other end of the spectrum and to be more or less ill. When none of the characteristics traditionally applied to health can be said to be enjoyed by the person, he/she is said to be hopelessly ill.

A reflection on what has been presented concerning the person, sickness, and health suggests that such a paradigm is not sufficient to illustrate the actual lived experience of the person. There are many aspects that make the person a whole being. The person has a body, personality, past and future, secret life, and a transcendent dimension. To become a whole, the person must also possess the ability to integrate these features into oneness; the person is an integrator who is able to bring the self into wholeness with the self and with the environment to which he/she relates. The purpose of this integration is to allow the person to pursue the human task of placing or discovering some order or meaning in his/her life.

The person can be said to enjoy good health when this integration takes place, when some balance has been achieved that allows for optimal functioning as a person in a particular state. A person can be said to be in poor health when this balance is lost, for whatever reason. When the person is not able to integrate the self with the self and/or with the environment, a condition of illness exists. The purpose of medical care, therefore, is to assist the person's effort to restore that balance, to arrive again at some integration of the self as a whole being, and once again to resume the human task.

In medical practice, this will mean different goals at different times for different people with different illnesses. Therefore, concern needs to be not only for *physical* life, but also for the unique and original *personal* life. I am speaking here of a quality of existence in which the individual has some meaningful self-awareness, other awareness, and capacity for interpersonal relationships and communication with the world. Health must have to do with this personal existence, which I will refer to as one's "quality of life."[34]

Quality of life does not mean that only a certain quality has any value, as if only productive life has quality. Quality is not something that can be determined quantitatively. Rather, quality has to do with the ability of the person, whether healthy or ill, to integrate his/her life and to be one with the self and with the world. A person does not need to have both legs, an excellent heart, or a great brain to be able to do this. Rather, one needs only the opportunity to restore and maintain the balance and meaning in life that makes one a whole person. In short, one needs some control within any life situation so that, with or without physical health, the person may be whole and integrated and able to pursue the human task of making life meaningful. This entails allowing the person to live as fully as he/she is able, to the full extent of his/her capabilities. For the sake of greater clarity, I will refer to this condition as "well-being," and reserve the word "health" to refer only to one's physical status. As such, health's opposite is "sickness."

The tentative definition put forward regarding health can now be replaced with the operative definition of this work for well-being: the state of being in which the individual does the best with the capacities he/she has and acts in ways that maximize those capacities to give personal significance and meaning. As such, the opposite of well-being is "suffering."

Based on this premise, I propose a more accurate paradigm than the traditional one—a paradigm of well-being. In this paradigm, the person is not on a linear continuum, but rather is within a multidimensional sphere. Lessened somewhat by a one-dimensional drawing, this paradigm might be visually presented as shown in Fig. 1.2.

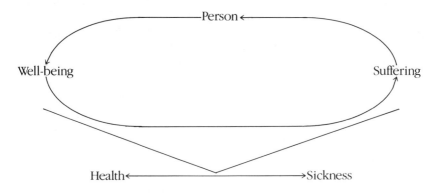

Fig 1.2 Paradigm of Well-Being

As in the more traditional paradigm, the person does move along a continuum between states of health and sickness. This, however, is not the primary movement of the person. Rather, the most fundamental movement is from suffering toward well-being. That is, it is the pursuit of the human task; the effort to integrate one's person and life into a meaningful whole so it can be lived; that is the most basic and fundamental activity of the human person.

As the person moves toward well-being, it is possible that the person may be healthy or ill. In either case, the person seeks to be an integrated whole, functioning in an optimal and meaningful way. The person is one with the self and the present situation, regardless of his/her health or sickness. The goal of the person is to live with an acceptable quality of life, as described earlier, even in the presence of apparent disabilities.

In the other direction, one may enjoy what could be described as good physical health yet be said to be suffering because of an inability to be whole and integrated. The person does not enjoy an acceptable quality of life because wholeness is somehow lacking. It could be said that the person is experiencing some threat with which he/she cannot cope at the moment.

Well-being has been defined as a state of wholeness in the person and the person's oneness with present life circumstances. Suffering is the antithesis. Suffering is a state of chaos in which a person is not at one with the self and/or with the environment. Further, suffering entails the fear that wholeness or integrity cannot or will not be restored, with the result being the destruction of the person. When this happens, the human task is disrupted, and life may appear to be meaningless.

Suffering is proposed as the antithesis to well-being because, although suffering is often equated with pain, it is actually much more than this physiological aspect. Pain and suffering are phenomenologically distinct.[35] Clinical experience prompts me to suggest that suffering is best defined as the perception that one is out of control in some aspect of personhood; integrity is threatened in such a way that the patient feels he/she is going to be destroyed as a person. This may involve physical pain, but it may be emotional as well. The instance of a woman whose cancer returned following the death of her husband illustrates this point. The woman was indeed suffering, but the suffering was not the cancer. Rather, the illness of cancer was in part caused by her suffering of abandonment and loneliness.

Cassel takes a similar approach:

> *Suffering occurs when an impending destruction of the person is perceived; it continues until the threat of disintegration has passed or until the integrity of the person can be restored in some other manner. . . . Most generally, suffering can be defined as the state of severe distress associated with events that threaten the intactness of the person.*[36]

When the person is suffering, he/she is experiencing some threat, which may or may not be physical, that appears to be more powerful than the person's own resources. If the person can begin to place or discover some order or meaning into what is happening, then the person will begin to move toward well-being. The crisis out of which the suffering arose may remain, but by becoming one again with the self and with what is happening, by placing or discovering some meaning in what is happening, the person is able to live out that life event. By resuming the human task, the suffering of chaos and meaninglessness yields to the order and meaning of well-being. The person is now well; not healthy perhaps, but well.

This paradigm responds to a need for a definition of health that includes weakness, age, and handicaps. It is possible to enjoy well-being but be weak because of heart trouble, well but be old and have difficulty getting around the house, and well but be handicapped and require a wheelchair for mobility. Each of these people can enjoy a sense of well-being because they are able, when given the chance, to be whole and integrated persons living meaningful lives. The person is not personally threatened by illness or physical limitations. What is important is the quality of life; that is, his/her being a whole person, able to live whatever is happening in a meaningful way. When the person is whole, there is a high quality of life. Physical attributes are secondary to total oneness. I hold that this applies equally to the person who is dying.

The goal of medical care must be to give the patient the greatest quality of life available. This is done by responding not only to the person's illness by treating a disease and its symptoms, but also, and more importantly, by responding to the person's suffering: the perception that one is out of control and that something will destroy the person. This can be done by allowing the person to be one with his/her present state, whether he/she is healthy or experiencing some acute, chronic, or terminal illness.

Quality of life will have different meanings for different people. For one experiencing some acute illness, it will include efforts to bring about a cure. For one who has a chronic illness, it will mean bringing about some modification of the body or life style in order to bring about a prolongation of life, as well as a response to whatever personal needs arise in these efforts. For the person who is terminally ill, quality of life will involve exercising some control within the dying event so that he/she may be one with the self as a dying person. The suffering of the dying is not so much in the act of dying as it is in being out of control of the dying. This, more often than not, is because people are not allowed to participate or find meaning in their own dying, sometimes because they are not allowed to die. If the person cannot pursue the human task of placing or discovering meaning in dying, he/she may never become an integrated and whole person who happens to be dying. The result is suffering even if there is no experience of physical pain, when the person could and should die in a state of well-being.

The next chapter will discuss how the person perceives a threat to personal integrity in illness. Chapter Three will explore the threats inherent in dying. By bringing together a discussion of how the person is threatened by sickness and death, it will be possible to show how those threats and the suffering they promote can be relieved so that the person can die well.

These will become the basis for a bioethical reflection on appropriate care for the dying.

NOTES

1. Maurice Reidy, *Foundations for a Medical Ethic: A Personal and Theological Exploration of the Ethical Issues in Medicine Today,* Veritas Publications, Dublin, 1978, p. 25.
2. Paul Ramsey, *The Patient as Person: Explorations in Medical Ethics,* Yale University Press, New Haven, 1970, p. 221.
3. Bernard Häring, *Medical Ethics,* Fides Publishers, Notre Dame, IN, 1973, p. 50.
4. See, for example, Joseph Fletcher, "Indicators of Humanhood: A Tentative Profile of Man," *The Hastings Center Report* 2, 1972, pp. 1-4; Louis Janssens, "Personalist Morals," *Louvain Studies* 3, 1970, pp. 5-16; Louis Janssens, "Norms and Priorities in a Love Ethic," *Louvain Studies* 6, 1977, pp. 207-238; Louis Janssens, "Artificial Insemination: Ethical Considerations," *Louvain Studies* 8, 1980, pp. 3-29; Paul Schotsmans, Faculteit Geneeskunde, Katholieke Universiteit Leuven, "Decision Making and Personal Conscience in Medical Care," unpublished paper, 1984; Michael Himes, "The Human Person in Contemporary Theologies: From Human Nature to Authentic Subjectivity," *Technological Powers and the Person,* ed. Albert S. Moraczewski et al., Pope John XXIII Medical-Moral Research & Education Center, St. Louis, 1983, pp. 288-312; Benedict M. Ashley, "An Integratd Christian View of the Human Person," *Technological Powers and the Person,* ed. Albert S. Moraczewski et al., Pope John XXIII Medical-Moral Research & Education Center, St. Louis, 1983, pp. 313-333; Benedict M. Ashley, *Theologies of the Body: Humanist and Christian,* Pope John XXIII Medical-Moral Research & Education Center, St. Louis, 1985, pp. 19-50; Häring, pp. 42-64.
5. Eric J. Cassel, "The Nature of Suffering and the Goals of Medicine," *The New England Journal of Medicine* 306, March 1982, pp. 630-645.
6. See O. Carl Simonton, Stephanie Matthews-Simonton, and James L. Creighton, *Getting Well Again: A Step-by-Step Self-Help Guide to Overcoming Cancer for Patients and Their Families,* Bantam Books, New York, 1978.
7. Cassel, p. 642.
8. Cassel, p. 643.
9. Cassel, p. 643.
10. Cassel, p. 643.
11. Cassel, p. 644.
12. Häring, p. 50.
13. Sharon L. Roberts, *Behavioral Concepts and the Critically Ill Patient,* Prentice-Hall, Englewood Cliffs, NJ, 1976, p. 75.
14. Roberts, p. 78.
15. Cassel, p. 644.
16. Robert J. Lifton and Eric Olson, *Living and Dying,* Bantam Books, New York, 1974.
17. Anne Munley, *The Hospice Alternative: A New Context for Death and Dying,* Basic Books, New York, 1983, p. 172.

18. Roberts, p. 97.
19. Paul Tillich, "The Meaning of Health," *Religion and Medicine,* ed. David R. Belgum, Iowa State University Press, Ames, IA, 1967, pp. 3-12.
20. See for example, Häring, p. 154; Abraham H. Maslow, *Toward a Psychology of Being,* 2nd ed., Van Nostrand Publishers, Princeton, NJ, 1968, p. 168; John G. Freymann, *The American Health Care System: Its Genesis and Trajectory,* Med Communications Publications, New York, 1974, p. 383; Henrick L. Blum, *Planning for Health: Development and Application of Social Change,* Behavioral Publishers, New York, 1974, p. 93; Benedict M. Ashley and Kevin D. O'Rourke, *Health Care Ethics: A Theological Analysis,* 2nd ed., Catholic Health Association of the United States, St. Louis, 1982, p. 25.
21. Los Angeles County–University of Southern California Cancer Center, *Psychological Aspects of Cancer,* LAC-USC Publication, Los Angeles, 1983, p. 17.
22. Tempkin Oswei, "The Scientific Approach of Disease: Specific Entity and Individual Sickness," *Scientific Changes,* ed. Alistair C. Crombie, Heinemann, London, 1963, pp. 629-660; Tempkin Oswei, "Health and Disease," *Dictionary of the History of Ideas,* vol. 2, ed. Philip P. Weiner, Charles Scribner's Sons, New York, 1973, pp. 395-407.
23. Arthur C. McGill, *Suffering: A Test of Theological Method,* Westminster Press, Philadelphia, 1982, pp. 20-37.
24. McGill, p. 22.
25. McGill, p. 28.
26. Jerry Falwell, "AIDS: The Judgement of God," *Liberty Report,* April 1987, p. 5.
27. Bede Griffiths, "Hinduism," *New Catholic Encyclopedia,* vol. VI, ed. William S. McDonald, McGraw-Hill, New York, 1967, pp. 1123-1136.
28. In another instance, a woman was headed for a temple to make an offering for her ill daughter. Her idea was that if the daughter was cursed, in which case a physician could do nothing, the offering would please the god, who would then lift the curse and allow the daughter to recover. If she did not get well, then the illness was not a curse, and they would seek medical assistance.
29. For a discussion of the difficulties associated with this term and a possible alternative, see Andrew Weil, *Health and Healing: Understanding Conventional and Alternative Medicine,* Houghton Mifflin, Boston, 1983, pp. 56-57.
30. Simonton et al., p. 27.
31. Elmer Green and Alyce Green, *Beyond Biofeedback,* Delacorte Press, New York, 1977.
32. Simonton et al., p. 27.
33. Ashley et al., p. 37.
34. The larger, moral debate of the "quality of life" within the context of the sanctity of life is not my concern here. Whereas the larger debate centers on the quality of life per se, I am concerned with the specific quality of a particular life at a given time and the attainment of the highest quality possible. In this, I take as a given that all life is sacred regardless of its relative quality at a given moment.
35. David Bakan, *Disease, Pain and Sacrifice: Toward a Psychology of Suffering,* Beacon Press, Chicago, 1971.
36. Cassel, p. 640.

2 / *An Understanding of Cancer and Aids*

The previous chapter discussed in some detail the significance of the person and what it means to present oneself as a patient. Chapter One also attempted to show that the person's well-being has to do not only with physical or mental health, but also with an overall integration of the person with the self and the world. How and to what extent physical health can be restored, as well as of what the person's well-being will consist, largely depend on the person's ability to cope with the particular threats involved. In this instance, those threats to personal integrity would flow from the nature of the disease.

To understand better how to relieve suffering and what wellness means to the person who is dying of cancer or acquired immune deficiency syndrome (AIDS), it is important to understand the threats inherent in each disease. The first section of this chapter, therefore, will focus on the nature of cancer and AIDS. The purpose will be to give a general overview of each disease so as to understand better their potential threat to the person.

The second section will look in greater detail at those threats as they are perceived by the patient. This will give insight into the direction medical care must take if it is to respond not only to the person's illness, but to the person's suffering as well.

The final section will deal with the coping mechanisms that cancer and AIDS patients use in dealing with disease. This is especially important because it will illustrate people's natural attempts to restore well-being by somehow regaining a sense of meaning and control within their lives. When this can be done, the person is able to move away from the perception of the impending destruction of their personhood. From this, it will be possible to draw some conclusions as to how medical care might assist in this process.

THE NATURE OF THE DISEASE

Cancer

The American Cancer Society (ACS) has made public education one of its chief goals so that people might be more aware of the dangers of cancer and the importance of early detection. To this end, they have established "seven warning signs" to alert people to the possibility of cancer:
1. Change in bowel or bladder habit
2. An open sore that does not heal
3. Unusual bleeding or discharge from any orifice
4. A thickening or lump in the breast or elsewhere
5. Indigestion or difficulty in swallowing
6. Recent change in a mole or wart
7. Persistent cough or hoarseness

Although these symptoms may indicate the possible presence of cancer, they do not indicate anything about cancer itself. To discover that, it is necessary to examine the pathology of a tumor.

Definition and Cause. A neoplasm, or tumor as it is more commonly known, consists of a mass of cells that have developed a permanent defect in their metabolism. That is, their structure and division activity have been permanently altered. This defect, which is passed on to other cells, causes the cells to grow in an abnormal, persistent, and excessive way.

A cancerous cell can perhaps best be described as a cell that has forgotten how to behave. Most normal cells divide at a given rate, multiply only within a specific locality, and stop when they meet dissimilar, adjacent tissue. Cancer cells, because of the metabolic defect, forget these rules of cellular growth. They divide faster, thus growing more quickly into a mass; they grow anywhere, thus allowing cancerous lung cells to grow in the liver; and they do not stop at adjacent tissue boundaries, but instead invade or compress surrounding tissues. There is a wide variety of cellular defects and behaviors, causing innumerable types of tumors that arise from essentially all bodily organs and tissues. The gestation period of a tumor is highly unpredictable, varying widely from a few weeks to several years. Once begun, the cellular growth rarely regresses without some form of treatment.

Tumors have many causes, some of which are proved experimentally, whereas others are theorized on presumptive evidence. Some causes are intrinsic to the person. These include heredity, age, sex, race, and an individual's hormonal and immunological status. When it is noted that every second approximately 10 million cells are produced in the body, one trillion every day, it is no wonder that something naturally goes wrong in the division of normal cells to bring about cancerous cells that have "forgotten" how to behave. Normally, the immune system is able to keep ahead of these defective cells. If the immune system is suppressed for some reason, such as with the presence of the AIDS virus, or if the defective cells are assisted by some hormonal imbalance, the body may no longer be able to care for itself in the prevention of the disease.

Other causes of cancer are extrinsic, including some chemicals and viruses, as well as solar and ionizing radiation. The exact cause of a particular tumor, however, cannot be easily determined. This is because only a small fraction of people exposed to a particular cause develop a specific type of tumor. Thus, in any one case, there are many potential causes.

Current theories suggest that the metabolic defect in the cells is the result of several factors, some of which merely initiate the defect and then disappear or no longer influence tumor growth. Once begun, continued growth is generally not dependent on the cause. Other factors seem to promote growth at a later time. Some tumors, even when substantially developed, remain dormant for extended periods until some new factor, either intrinsic or extrinsic to the person, stimulates it to further growth. Some have suggested that these factors include those of an emotional nature.

Historically, attempts have been made to define a connection between cancer and human emotions. Galen, a physician in the second century AD, first observed that a cheerful woman was less inclined to have cancer than a woman who had a depressed nature. In 1701, Gendron wrote a paper on the connection between the difficulties in life and the incidence of cancer. In 1822, Nunn spoke of a woman with a tumor that had apparently been in remission until the shock of her husband's death. The tumor then began to grow again, and she died.

In 1926, Evan published a study of 100 cancer patients. She showed that many of these patients had lost a significant relationship before their diagnosis was made.[1] She found, too, that many of these people had invested their identity in another person, job, or role, rather than developing their own individuality. When this other person died, or when a job was lost or a role significantly changed, the person was left with no sense of identity. She also found that many of these people consistently put another's needs ahead of their own.

LeShan reported findings similar to Evan's in 1977.[2] He mentions four typical components apparent in the life histories of 76 percent of the more than 500 cancer patients interviewed:

1. The person's youth was marked by feelings of isolation, neglect, and despair, with intense interpersonal relationships being difficult and often perceived as dangerous.
2. In early childhood, the person had been able to establish a strong relationship with another or later had found great personal satisfaction in his/her vocation. The person then went on to put tremendous energy into this relationship or role, such that it became the focus of his/her life.
3. The relationship was ended or the role taken away, resulting in despair and often awakening the past pains of difficulty in relationships or in self-confidence.
4. One of the most fundamental characteristics of these patients was that they kept their despair and disappointment to themselves, unable to express pain or anger with or toward others.

The debate concerning the role that emotions play in the development and prognosis of cancer has growth in recent years.[3] The work of people such as Boyd, Cousins, and Weil suggests a strong link between cancer, or illness in general, and human emotions.[4] Other studies, such as that done by Cassileth et al., argue that any seemingly apparent link is more of a myth than a reality.[5] Although the debate certainly calls for more research, present information does suggest that the connection is not to be dismissed out of hand. It may be more a question of discovering the nature of the connection and the degree of the influence rather than determining its existence.

Natural History of Progressive Tumor Growth. There are three phases in the natural history of progressive tumor growth: (1) subclinical, (2) clinically early, and (3) clinically advanced disease. Each will be examined briefly, with particular attention paid to the third, since this is the clinical phase of the terminally ill.

Subclinical. Unless the tumor is located superficially, it will not be clinically detectable at this phase, usually being detectable only after an appropriate screening test. The tumor is likely to be within a small, local area, although invasion into nearby tissues and metastasis to other parts of the body may have already begun.

Clinically early. At this phase, an uncertain percentage of people with cancer will have occult or unknown metastases. Exactly how many and where will vary according to the type or primary tumor. Most people seek medical attention at this stage.

Clinically advanced. In the clinically advanced patient, there is usually widespread disease, with the total mass of tumor cells amounting to about two pounds. Specific reference to the amount of tumor growth gives insight into the inability of radical surgery, radiation, and chemotherapy to bring about a total and complete remission. The high incidence of progressive failure and recurrence is why cancer patients are often said to be "clinically free" rather than cured of cancer. Referral to the mass of tumor involved also gives some insight into the rationale for the eventual shift in therapy from control of the disease to control of symptoms, as in palliative care.

When a person presents him/herself for care at this phase, the primary tumor has most often been treated previously, and there is generally no evidence of its presence. Instead, the person appears with metastatic disease. In other cases, the primary tumor may still be present, although it is almost always accompanied by metastases. In cases where the primary tumor is present, the person in a clinically advanced phase may have been negligent in care of the tumor. This is sometimes the case with cancer of the breast, cervix, vulva, and skin. In these instances, the primary tumor may appear as a large, fungating mass. At other times, the tumor may be present because it was unresponsive to treatment. Most often, however, the presence of the primary tumor is caused by a posttreatment local recurrence. When this is the case, the tumor is generally regarded as one manifestation of a more generalized metastatic disease. This is often seen with cancer of the breast, head, or neck. Local recurrence is virtually certain if the tumor is not completely removed during initial treatment.

Because the person who is dying with cancer is generally in a clinically advanced phase of the disease and is therefore most often troubled with metastatic disease, it is important to discuss metastatic cancer in more detail.

Metastatic cancer. Most carcinomas, as well as some melanomas and neuroblastomas, metastasize by spreading as a single cell or clump of cells to the nearest group of lymph nodes. If the clump is large enough, it can cause an obstruction in the flow of lymphatic fluids. This results in a discoloration of the skin, often referred to as the "peau d'orange" effect in cases of breast cancer.

Once established in the lymph nodes, these tumor cells continue to multiply and soon begin to replace the normal structure of the lymph node. Any new tumor cells that move into this node are deflected to others. In most cases, this happens according to an orderly pattern that is anatomically predictable. As the lymph node is replaced by the metastatic tumor, it usually becomes enlarged and can cause discomfort as a result of pressure exerted on the surrounding tissue. Large, superficial lymph node metastases sometimes ulcerate through the skin.

There is a wide variation of characteristics involved with metastases. For example, it is clinically common for malignant tumors to vary in their capacity to metastasize. Gliomas, on the one hand, are fatal because they invade locally within the central nervous system (CNS); distant metastases of gliomas, however, are almost unknown. On the other hand, other tumors disseminate widely throughout the body; it is not known why this occurs. The number, size, and distribution of metastatic tumors will also vary. It is important to stress, however, that this is not a random occurrence. There are definite sites of preference. Although certain tissues and organs are regularly involved by metastases some primary tumors appear to metastasize preferentially to certain sites. At the same time, some tissues, such as the spleen and striated muscles, appear to be naturally resistant to tumor growth.

There is also evidence that metastases at different locations in the same person may grow at different rates and differ in their response to radiation and chemotherapy. For example, in the case of a primary tumor of the breast, a metastasis to the bone sometimes responds well to treatment, whereas metastases to soft tissues are generally unresponsive. Wherever the site, metastatic growth is almost always progressive. It is the exception when the progressive growth rate of the disease declines. This is true even when there is a partial or complete remission, which itself is almost always temporary.

The extent of metastases in cancer patients is often underestimated. Autopsy reports show that, in any one patient, there is always a certain amount of metastatic disease that has gone undetected.[6] This is significant in that most fatal cancers result in death because of the primary tumor metastasizing to another location. It is rare that death is directly related to the presence of the primary tumor.

It is sometimes assumed that the clinical diagnosis of cancer follows an orderly progression of primary tumor followed eventually by some metastases. Several variations in this pattern, however, may develop. The disease may first become clinically apparent at the site of the metastases rather than as a primary tumor. In addition, the time between identification of the primary tumor and development of metastases varies. Clinical experience indicates that the metastatic process is often underway by the time the person seeks medical attention for what is believed to be a local tumor. On the other hand, as many as 15 or 20 years may pass before any metastases become apparent. The reasons for this variation are unknown.

Acquired Immune Deficiency Syndrome (AIDS)

AIDS was first identified in the United States in June 1981. At that time, the Centers for Disease Control (CDC) in Atlanta noted an unusual increase in requests for development of a new drug to treat *Pneumocystis carinii* pneumonia (PCP). Further investigation led to the discovery that this increased incidence and greater difficulty in treating PCP was primarily among male homosexuals whose immune system had become severely depressed for unknown reasons.

It was also noticed that some of these patients also had lesions associated with Kaposi's sarcoma, a form of cancer usually found with older men. When this information was put together with the fact that, in major cities across the United States, young homosexual men had been dying of Kaposi's sarcoma since 1978, the CDC authorities knew they were presented with a new and virile disease.

Definition and Transmission. Two independent teams in the United States and France isolated the AIDS virus in 1983. In the United States, the research team of the National Cancer Institute (NCI) isolated a virus that it designated as the *human T-lymphotropic virus type III (HTLV-III)*, so named because of the destructive effect of the virus on the T lymphocytes.[7] At the Pasteur Institute in France, scientists classified this same virus as the *lymphadenopathy-associated virus (LAV)*. The virus is also commonly referred to as the *human immunodeficiency virus (HIV)*. This is the term that will be used here.

There are many myths associated with the transmission of HIV. A 1987 survey of the National Center for Health Statistics indicates that 25 percent of the people in the United States believe that AIDS is transmitted by donating blood. Other misconceptions include 38 percent who believe it can be contracted through mosquitoes and other insects, and 31 percent who fear they may catch the virus through the use of a public toilet.[8] It is now known, however, that HIV is transmitted only through the direct contact of one's own blood with infected blood, blood products, or body fluids. The primary means of transmission, therefore, are considered to be sexual, particularly anal, intercourse and intravenous (IV) drug use.

In the case of drugs, the virus may enter a person's blood when a contaminated needle is inserted into a vein. During sexual intercourse, it is believed that tiny, imperceptible tears occur in the vagina, anus, or along the penis during penetration. This probably occurs more readily and often in the anus because of its more sensitive lining, thus explaining why the virus has spread so quickly among homosexual men. The virus, present in the semen or vaginal fluids, may enter the blood through these tears.

Although it is true that the virus has also been found to be present in other body fluids such as saliva and tears, this is rare and its transmission through these fluids has not been proved.[9] Nevertheless, oral sex with an infected person may still put one at risk, particularly if semen is taken into the mouth. Any cuts or irritations of the mouth or gums may allow the virus to enter the blood. The pattern of HIV transmission has been shown in the United States to be most often from men to men and men to women, and less frequently from women to men, and women to women.

Although HIV was first diagnosed among male homosexuals and IV drug users, it has spread through the general population through sexual contact and transfusions of blood that were infected by the virus before its discovery and before screening tests were available. As of Sept. 1, 1987, 41,250 cases of AIDS had been reported to the CDC. This group consisted of:

65%	Homosexually or bisexually oriented males
17%	IV drug users
8%	Homosexually oriented males using IV drugs
4%	Heterosexually oriented males and females
2%	As a result of a blood transfusion with infected blood
1%	Hemophiliac persons who received infected blood
3%	No immediately identifiable cause[10]

It should be noted that the danger of exposure to HIV through a blood transfusion today is extremely unlikely since the development in March 1985 of the enzyme-linked immunosorbent assay (ELISA) test kits to determine the presence of AIDS antibodies in blood. According to Fisher, "voluntary deferment and screening of all donors has virtually eliminated the risk of AIDS or HIV infection following blood transfusion."[11]

HIV can also be transmitted in vivo from mother to child. Transmission may result from transplacental passage, intrapartum exposure to infected maternal blood, or through postnatal exposure to breast milk.[12] A 1987 study of Kings County Hospital Center in New York suggests that as many as 2 percent of all women giving birth in major cities in the United States may be infected with HIV.[13] A 1986 update of the CDC revealed that, of 231 cases of AIDS in children under 13 years of age, 76 percent had been born to mothers who were infected with HIV. Another 5 percent were hemophiliac children who received infected blood, 14 percent included children who had received a blood transfusion, and 5 percent were of no immediately identifiable risk group. Of these, 58 percent developed PCP. Only 4 percent developed Kaposi's sarcoma, which seems to be found principally among male homosexuals who develop AIDS. A large number of these children developed chronic lymphocytic interstitial pneumonitis, a condition unique to children who develop AIDS.[14]

The *Surgeon General's Report* published in 1986 estimates that approximately 1.5 million people in the United States have been exposed to HIV and are capable of transmitting it to others.[15] The actual figure, however, may be much higher. The majority of people with AIDS in the United States became infected between 1981 and 1982, but it is now known that some people may have been infected as early as 1979.[16] Several hospitals in the United States are now testing samples of blood given in transfusions before 1981 to better determine who may be at risk.

Not everyone who has been exposed to HIV will actually develop AIDS. However, even if an infected person does not, he/she is still capable of transmitting the virus to others through sexual contact or contact with body fluids and another's blood.

Some people who are exposed to the virus may develop *AIDS-related complex (ARC)*. ARC is a condition in which the person tests positive for HIV and develops a specific set of clinical symptoms that are generally less severe than those associated with AIDS. These may include a loss of appetite, weight loss, fever, night sweats, skin rashes, diarrhea, tiredness, lack of resistance to infection, or swollen lymph nodes. These are also the symptoms of other diseases, so ARC may be difficult to diagnose.

Of those who are infected with the AIDS virus, the surgeon general predicts that approximately 20 to 30 percent will develop AIDS within five years.[17] This figure may vary significantly from place to place depending on the population of the risk groups in a specific area. It is estimated that by 1991, there will be some 270,000 cases of AIDS in the United States, resulting in some 179,000 deaths.[18]

HIV Replication Cycle. AIDS is a condition brought on by the presence of the human retrovirus HIV in one's blood. On entering the blood, the virus attacks the T_4 helper lymphocytes, the mediator cells of the immune system. Once inside the lymphocyte, the virus sheds its protective protein coat, exposing the core of the virus containing ribonucleic acid (RNA). The virus uses what is known as a reverse transcriptase to translate the invading RNA into deoxyribonucleic acid (DNA). This allows the virus to be inserted into the chromosomes of the host cell in preparation for reproduction. When this happens, seroconversion takes place. That is, the body begins to produce antibodies to fight off the infection. These antibodies, sometimes referred to as AIDS antibodies, can usually be detected in the blood two weeks to three months after infection. In rare cases, the AIDS antibodies may not become evident until six months after exposure. Once a person is exposed to HIV, it appears likely that the person is infected for life.

HIV multiplies by budding from the surface of the T_4 cells, which are eventually destroyed in the process. As the disease progresses, the infected cell becomes a "factory" for the production of other infected cells. As more and more T_4 cells are destroyed, the immune system fails. This results in the person being left vulnerable to a host of opportunistic diseases, diseases that could otherwise be controlled by the body's natural defenses. These include various infections, cancers, and neurological disorders. Because of

31

its devastating effect on the immune system, AIDS is generally considered to be fatal.

HIV Classification. Tuazon and Labriola have classified the possible manifestations of HIV infection into four categories.[19] These show the wide spectrum of signs and symptoms that may arise as a result of exposure to the virus.

Acute infection. Citing a 1985 study by Cooper et al., Tuazon and Labriola speak of this category as including those people infected with HIV who experience transient symptoms similar to, for example, those of acute mononucleosis. These symptoms most often become apparent at the time of infection or shortly thereafter. In Cooper's study, no treatment was initiated, and the patients recovered spontaneously.

Asymptomatic infection. A significant number of people infected with HIV will experience no symptoms of infection. In these cases, the only indication of HIV is the presence of the AIDS antibody in the blood.

Generalized lymphadenopathy. Some people infected with HIV will experience persistent and generalized complications associated with the lymph nodes. This condition is defined by the presence, for at least six months, of nodes of at least 1 cm in diameter in at least two noncontiguous, extrainguinal sites.[20] Most people who experience this condition will be asymptomatic or will experience only mild symptoms such as a low-grade fever. Abrams et al. estimate that each year 1 percent of those in this category will develop AIDS.[21]

Other diseases. This last category includes all symptoms other than those involving the lymphatic system. These include an unexplained fever that persists over a month, a weight loss of greater than 10 percent, and unexplained diarrhea for over a month.

Neurological complications have also been associated with HIV infection. These may include, but are not limited to, impaired concentration and a mild memory loss that may progress to severe impairment. A typical late development in patients with AIDS is severe dementia, with a computed tomography (CT) scan showing cerebral atrophy.[22]

The majority of AIDS cases involve the presence of some opportunistic infection. These include some forms of pneumonia, meningitis, or encephalitis. These will be discussed in more detail in Chapter Four, which will focus on various therapies in palliative care.

CANCER AND AIDS AS A THREAT TO THE PERSON

The greatest threat to anyone is the threat of the destruction of personhood, that sense that one is going to be overwhelmed by an invading force over which the person has no control. In the preceding chapter's paradigm for well-being, this sense of impending destruction and personal chaos was referred to as suffering. It has also been called an "internal hopelessness."[23] This suffering is rooted in a loss of control over one's ability to integrate the characteristics of the person into a wholeness of being. This section will examine how cancer and AIDS pose such a threat to the person by examining the effects of the disease and the disease process on the person's body image, sense of independence, environment, relationships, and self-worth.[24]

Body Image

All persons exist within a body and relate in and through that body to the self and the surrounding world. In relating to the self, the body offers the person a framework within which to exist. The body gives the person capacities and abilities with which to work and grow in personhood. The person develops a self-image through this process. By coming to know and understand the body, the person comes to know and understand much about the self and to depend on the body for continued self-expression. Likewise, in relating to the world, the person communicates and acts through the body to integrate the self into the community in a meaningful way. The person needs the body as a vehicle for relating, and uses it to establish and maintain social relationships. The body is thus a frame of reference for the person. When the frame of reference is changed, the person is changed as well:

> *To lose or be threatened with the loss of a complex, co-ordinated and controlled functional activity which has been achieved and integrated into the personal system is to lose or be threatened with the loss of self. Psychosocially, the loss, or the threat of loss, of self is equivalent to loss of life.[25]*

At the onset of an illness, the person has a sense that the whole self is fighting the disease. If recovery follows, that sense is preserved. When an illness persists and the prognosis becomes less favorable, the person begins to view the disease as having the upper hand.[26] The person begins to believe that the body is no longer controlled by him/herself, but by the disease. The disease decides where the person can go, when and for how long, what the person can eat and drink, and even with whom and in what manner the person may relate. Strauss speaks of this as a betrayal on the part of the body toward the person.[27] Because the body has once betrayed the person, it may do so again at any time. With few exceptions, most people who are dying with cancer have had a long struggle with disease and therapy, whereas those with AIDS have seen their body deteriorate with what is sometimes described as frightening speed. The sense of betrayal with both is strong. This may be particularly true among AIDS patients, whose condition is, by definition, one of constant physical vulnerability.

Another concept suggested by Roberts is that every person has a mental image of appearance.[28] This image may or may not correspond to reality. Whether or not the perception is accurate is not significant. What is significant is that the perception determines behavior and influences one's self-image. Illness brings about changes in one's body and therefore in one's self-perception. If someone believes, for example, that he/she is able to relate to the world principally through musical talents, the loss of the tonal quality of one's voice will threaten the perception of the self. A case from a lived experience is more telling:

> *I loved running. It was my whole life. I'd go to school, go to work, but track was everything. I was only eighteen, and the coach was encouraging me. So when they told me I might never run again, man, I just didn't want to live anymore.*[29]

The person must adjust, must return to some sense of wholeness that allows the person's integrity to remain intact in spite of the changes. Roberts calls this "adaptation." Adaptation to any change in the body's function or structure:

> *. . . depends upon the nature of the threat, its meaning to the critically ill patient, his coping ability, the response from others significant to him, and the assistance available to him and his family as changes occur. With the occurrence of any injury or illness, the individual finds himself thrown into experiences that force him to alter his concept of self and body image.*[30]

Adaptation depends not only on the nature of the threat, but also on the perception of the threat. In fact, more often than not, it is one's perception of a threat that will determine the response. As Corbeil points out, "The quality of disturbance is much more related to the individual's perception of it than to the actual fact."[31]

The perception of changes in a person's body image can be particularly disturbing in cases of AIDS because of the rapidity of those changes. It is not unusual for people who are self-conscious to scrutinize others for some reaction to their appearance.[32] Others express concerns that initiating new relationships will be hampered, as well as fears that family members, especially children, will be frightened by the sudden changes in appearance.

Physical changes common among AIDS patients include extreme weight loss, skin discoloration, disfigurement by tumors, and loss of hair. Because a small pimple or bruise might be the sign of more serious trouble, some AIDS patients become obsessed with examining their bodies for signs of new lesions.[33] Frierson and Lippmann report that patients with depression have the poorest self-image, which is often out of proportion to their actual appearance.

Although in cases of AIDS, body changes tend to be quite rapid, with cancer they may take longer to develop. As illness continues to pervade the body and take its toll, gradual and less dramatic changes may appear that begin to drain the person's resources and self-image. For example, one young man was diagnosed as having acute lymphoblastic leukemia. After five weeks of chemotherapy, which resulted in the remission of the disease, he began a two- to three-year course of treatment aimed at total eradication. In the first phase of treatment, he described himself as looking at life as a survivor from a concentration camp:

In that short period of time, I lost all feeling of self-worth and self-confidence. I was just a bag of bones, a burden on everyone, stripped of any feeling of self-esteem. Physical energy is easier to replace than emotional psychic energy, and it took a long time to regenerate mine, even after my physical condition began to improve.[34]

When these physical changes are clearly visible, they may prevent the person's easy return to former ways of living, thus demanding new ways of approaching personal, interpersonal, and social aspects of life. As one woman who had a mastectomy stated, "People always want to know which is your 'bad side.' "

Disfigurement is not the only threat posed to the body. The steady loss of bodily function is also a constant reminder of the continued progress of the disease and the failure of the body. It might begin with a restriction of activity, leading next to one's ability to move about freely. Finally, one loses control over even one's own bodily functions, such as with incontinence. Indeed, as Roberts writes:

Loss of body functions has overwhelming implications to critical care patients. An individual's body is anchored to his need for self-esteem. Any body alteration disturbs his integrity and appears to be a movement down the negative continuum toward death.[35]

This can be especially true with the loss of sexual function, since very often people place a high expectation on themselves as sexual beings. In the case of a mastectomy, one woman awoke from surgery to learn that the surgeon had performed a modified mastectomy, being careful to perform it in such a way that she would still be able to wear sleeveless, low-cut dresses. She responded angrily, insisting that she was concerned about her health, not her looks. She later admitted that this was the reaction of her "wounded self." That her sexual appearance was important is expressed in her words of gratitude toward her husband: "He kept me feeling like a woman."[36] Men, too, will experience a loss of self over the onset of sterility or impotence associated with continued weakening. The inability of lack of opportunity to respond sexually may also carry the burden of a perceived failure toward one's sexual partner, adding to a loss of self-respect.[37]

The aspect of sexuality plays a significant role in the self-imaging of people with AIDS. Because of its common and inappropriate association with homosexuality, the reality that one is infected with HIV often raises serious questions of self-identity for oneself and others. Heterosexually oriented persons, for example, have felt compelled to emphasize their use of drugs to avoid an association with what may be considered to be a less respectable identity. Also, because of the relative youth of those most often afflicted with AIDS, many who become infected have not yet resolved developmental issues concerning identity. One man, for example, had expressed conflict over his sexual preference in his life and at first experienced relief that, after his diagnosis of AIDS, he could "avoid sexuality." His frequent thoughts of suicide, however, indicate how impossible avoiding one's sexuality can be, especially in the light of a fatal illness that, for him, was tied directly to living out that sexuality.[38] Because of the stigma often associated with AIDS, even people who have been secure in their own sexual identity often find themselves reassessing themselves and past behavior.

The identification of AIDS as some form of divine punishment also may have an impact on a person's sexuality. Guilt, even among those who have demonstrated a degree of healthy self-adjustment, is not uncommon. A reassessment of one's religious beliefs also may occur. Further, once one knows that he/she is HIV positive, any further sexual activity becomes extremely dangerous to potential partners, forcing many to deny their diagnosis and endanger others or to withdraw from the affection they have enjoyed. Fear of contracting AIDS from another may also move people into an isolation they do not desire and for which they are not prepared. Many persons with AIDS report that they have not been touched or held affectionately since their diagnosis and thus have not experienced an important source of comfort and acceptance.[39]

The pain that often accompanies changes in the body is a constant reminder of a life controlled by disease. Medication can ease pain, but even medication is a reminder of the loss of a healthy body. Used regularly and on schedule, it is often possible to live reasonably free of discomfort. As Munley points out, however, although the person may intellectually accept that with a strict schedule and the correct amount of medicine, pain can be controlled, emotionally there can be a sense that chemical substances now exercise more power over the person's life than the person does.[40] This perception may grow as the dose needed to control the pain increases. In addition, one can become emotionally dependent on medication to maintain health. As one patient whose cancer went into remission said:

> *For years, I had yearned for the last day of chemotherapy. But when it happened, I was scared down to my very soul. I had suddenly lost my crutch. As much as I hated taking the drugs, as much as I couldn't wait for it to be over, it was a sort of insurance policy. It kept me well.[41]*

Each person who experiences some alteration to the body will feel the threat of being found to be inadequate or unattractive as a person. Each person will perceive this threat differently, since it is also related to the extent the individual's patterns of adaptation are interrupted. All people develop patterns of behavior that meet personal needs for security. Some of these may depend entirely on certain bodily functions or organs. If these organs or their functioning become disrupted or are lost because of disease, the threat to the person is perceived as being greater than if an unimportant function or organ is disrupted, even if the disease were to be more life threatening.

Independence

Illness poses a series of threats to a person's independence and ability to exercise some control within one's life direction. Independence can be defined as the expectancy or probability held by a person that his/her behavior will lead to the accomplishment of certain personally chosen goals. The opposite of this is powerlessness: the perceived lack of personal and/or internal control within certain events in certain situations. As one person with AIDS described it:

> *This is a very uncooperative illness for people who like to have their lives scheduled. There's a sudden explosiveness that doesn't allow you to predict, to plan.[42]*

Disease is not the only threat to a person's independence. There is also a perceived loss of control to machines and to the people who operate them. A 1980 study involving patients receiving chemotherapy offers some interesting insights.[43]

In this study of 33 patients, only three sought a second opinion after receiving a diagnosis of cancer. The overwhelming majority perceived themselves as dependent on the judgment of the physician and were therefore unlikely to question any medical recommendations by seeking outside advice. In addition, some gave the impression that they would go anywhere for therapy, regardless of how they were treated by the medical team. One patient is quoted as saying: "I have to be satisfied; my doctor put me here."[44]

Other studies have shown that often there is a reluctance on the part of patients to make demands on medical staff, particularly demands for more personal attention, out of fear of retribution. A powerlessness and subsequent dependence emerge out of this situation in which the person believes that he/she is not free to express concerns for personal therapy. These fears of possible retribution are often symptomatic of the person's feelings of powerlessness and of an inability to cope.

The person who becomes a patient often has no control over how he/she will be handled during treatment and senses a loss of control over how others relate to him/her. In other settings, one is free to allow or not allow a certain closeness or distance in relationships. That authority is lost in illness. For one elderly woman, being addressed by her first name, rather than as "Mrs." and her last name, was "a terrible experience." She was powerless over the manner in which others related to her. Further, the person in a healthcare setting must permit his/her body to be handled and manipulated. Often, patients describe the conducting of tests or receiving of care as acts by which they feel "violated" or "raped."

This experience of powerlessness can be aggravated by a lack of information concerning the illness or the treatment. As one patient stated, "You can't fight something unless you know what it is."[45] A lack of information is often unintentional on the part of the medical staff, being instead the result of necessarily hurried or highly technical explanations. Intentional or not, the result is the same: a lack of knowledge.

The amount and kind of information a patient receives are of great importance, especially in view of the general holistic approach taken in this book and in the individual's increasing sense of responsibility for his/her illness and health. Some research has suggested that the way a person seeks and uses information regarding illness may play a role in the survival of some patients.[46]

A sense of powerlessness is often present in cases of AIDS as a result of the relative youth of the person involved. Many people with AIDS find themselves hospitalized for the first time with some complication brought on as a result of the suppression of the immune system. The combination of youth and inexperience with sickness or a hospital setting can compound feelings of powerlessness. Antisocial patients, for example, may rebel against this situation and become management problems. Frierson and Lippmann write that, in cases where AIDS patients seek to leave a hospital against medical advice, an attempt by the person to regain some control is often the issue. On the other end of the spectrum, depressed patients sometimes regress and become totally dependent on care givers.[47] It has also been shown that children or young adults who have become infected as a result of a blood transfusion often suffer from a tendency toward overprotectiveness on the part of their parents.[48]

Because AIDS leaves a person vulnerable to many infections, some people express the frustration that they are at the mercy of anyone with a cold. Feelings of powerlessness have also been shown to develop as a result of parental efforts to use the illness as an excuse to exercise greater authority. In severe cases, feelings of helplessness are sometimes heightened by the inability of the person to care for him/herself, prompting one patient to attempt suicide in order to at least be able "to decide when I die."[49]

All persons, therefore, want to maintain an element of power or control within themselves and their environment. When illness forces the individual to relinquish that control to a disease, machines, or to others, he/she may experience an overwhelming sense of powerlessness. It may be safe to state that the more acute the situation or the person's illness, the more powerless the person is likely to feel.

Environment

A person's wholeness depends not only on the private resources of the self, but also on interaction with the environment. Each person is aware of the environment to one extent or another and has a certain amount of control within it. Part of this involves the person's openness to outside stimuli. When most people have had enough, they are generally able to simply shut out any more information. Part of the way in which people integrate life is through this ability to control receptivity to stimuli. The person cannot always stop the stimuli but can exercise some control over its reception.

The person who is ill loses much of that control, especially if the person requires hospitalization in an acute care setting. Placed in a setting of strange people and strange machines, the person's world is transformed from a friendly home to a foreign and often frightening place. The person has no control over where he/she will be placed or with whom he/she will have to deal. Further, the person will have no control over stimuli. Sounds and sights will shower in on the person continuously and often without permission. Roberts calls this a case of "environmental overdose":

> *The environmental overdose of the critically ill patient may not seem as immense as it does to the city dweller, but we must remember that the physically healthy city dweller is able to change his environment, whereas the patient is a captive member of his environment. It must also be remembered that illness alters an individual's perceptions. He may no longer be able to differentiate meaningful stimuli because the sounds are all new or foreign to him. In our desire to assist our patient, we only create an environment that is too much, too soon, too fast. The patient is then subjected to the world of environmental overdose or sensory overload.[50]*

This overdose is partly caused by the orientation of the care setting, with which the person, particularly if young, may not be familiar. People go into a care setting because of some trauma that demands immediate attention. The setting is established to meet the immediate health needs of the person. Because of this, the setting is not always able to respond to the personal needs of the person. Although this may be an efficient way to run an acute care setting, there can be a danger in losing sight of the ultimate purpose of care: the well-being of the whole person. It is important that the medical profession consider the more personal needs of the person as well as the specific therapy necessitated by the illness or trauma.

One difficulty faced by the person is trying to become oriented to the new and constantly changing surroundings. This orientation often takes place while a nurse is giving a series of instructions, which may include an order not to get up alone. In many cases, the patient will get up out of bed alone simply because visually taking in all there is to see and hearing all there is to hear is often just too much, too quickly. The person is neither stupid nor obstinate, merely disoriented in an environment within which little, if any, control may be exercised.

Another reason for the person's disorientation is the intensity of the care environment. This may often increase the person's anxiety over being ill. Machines often add to the intensity of this anxiety. In spite of their necessary lifesaving functions and reassuring qualities to some, these devices are often perceived as threatening to others. They become ideal objects on which to project anger and fear.

Many people, because of their ability to both hear and watch monitors, are likely to attempt to assess their condition from signs in the environment. The environment dictates, to some extent, what the person thinks of his/her condition. The information received and the conclusions reached may be inaccurate and, in some circumstances, frightening.

In short, the person in the care setting often experiences a loss of control within his/her environment. Although all that occurs in the care setting may facilitate the cure of an illness, the person will, initially at least, suffer from a sense of being out of control within one's world.

Relationships

A person's ability to relate may also be threatened through illness. The result is that many patients experience loneliness.

When someone is ill, some separation from others is usually involved. This is necessitated by many factors. Often the one who is ill merely needs to be alone to rest. At other times, the disease will be contagious and require some period of isolation. In these instances, the person is alone but may not be lonely. Hoskisson expresses this in writing that sometimes people are aware of their aloneness and at other times they are not.[51] The distinction between these two states is found in the awareness of a need for contact and the ability to attain it. Hoskisson states:

> *Loneliness is the conscious experience of separation from something or someone desired, required, or needed. It is not solitariness, for there the separation is not felt, nor is it a lack of physical or social contact, for as we all know the presence of people does not assuage it. So there must be experienced a need, a desire for contact, and an inability to make it.*[52]

Roberts calls the awareness of the need and desire for contact and the inability to experience it as the "loneliness of psychological pain."[53] This loneliness is often especially painful for one with AIDS, which often presents the person with the possibility of rejection by those closest to him/her. AIDS often carries the stigma of an association to behavior with which many are not comfortable. In addition, people are frightened of others with AIDS, not simply because it may be contagious, but because they perceive it as being so mysterious and deadly. This aspect of loneliness occurs when the person must be away or is separated from significant other persons.

Being separated from others has the obvious effect of causing one to be alone. Loneliness is part of this experience because the person finds him/herself left to personal resources in the face of the unknown. Sometimes when most physically challenged or weakened, a person who is ill may find him/herself also dealing with isolation and loss. The person may feel weak, unsupported and distanced from a community where values, ideals, and faith were fostered and shared.

Even when the community is nearby, the person may feel alone in the experience. The person has a keen awareness that no one else knows what he/she is going through, how much it hurts, and what it is like to have this disease. This belief that others cannot understand because they do not share in the experience can keep the person alone in the presence of others.

Finally, when the person feels alone, there is no opportunity to relate through his/her body. Most often, the only possible experience of relating is that of receiving. There is little, if any, opportunity to give. This lack of reciprocal relationships can result in the person's feeling separated from oneself. Without the ability to relate bodily, the person may take on a perspective similar to that often held by others and watch as a body, but not a person, receives attention.

The environment of care can contribute to feelings of loneliness. Natural relationships are not part of the hospital scene. Rather, relationships are based on the roles that patients, nurses, and physicians are each expected to fulfill, following set rules of conduct and modes of behavior. The person is also in a system that is alien and can easily make one feel that one "doesn't belong" to what is happening. Indeed, any care setting has an order and runs as efficiently as possible. This is the institution's order, however, not the person's. Loneliness may result.

Although it can be said that the patient is the most important person in the healthcare facility, activity sometimes suggests otherwise. In this activity, there is a hint that the patient will be forgotten, a suggestion reinforced when no one comes to answer the bed bell. A publication of the Los Angeles County–University of Southern California Cancer Center lists one of the major fears of cancer patients as the fear of being abandoned by their physician.[54] This is an even greater fear among some than is the fear of dying. As Dunphy points out:

> *Finally, and most important of all . . . the patient is not afraid of death, but he is terribly afraid of being abandoned by his physician in the face of death.*[55]

The fear of abandonment is illustrated in the person's thoughts on the characteristics of the ideal physician. In Bean's study, these characteristics were identified as compassionate, reassuring, understanding, open, and warm.[56] In short, the ideal physician was viewed as someone who is committed to meeting the social and emotional needs of the patient, helping him/her to grow in a sense of security that will help ward off feelings of loneliness. Simonton et al. refer to this as "expertise that cares."[57]

Blaney writes that the two primary aspects of mental healthcare needed by a person with AIDS are the information and support that the medical profession can offer.[58]

A young man hospitalized for bone cancer tells how important the relationship with his physician and the others on the healthcare staff were to him:

> *The doctor stayed with me in my room for about an hour, talking to me, keeping my spirits up. If it hadn't been for him, I would never have made it that night.*[59]

Referring to the nurse who prepared him for surgery to amputate his leg, the same man remarked:

> *He'd been shaving my leg, just breezing along, but then he started shaving it real slow, taking extra care like he didn't want to hurt it no more, giving it all respect like it was going to stay with me. I was feeling him caring so much for me. It's having the caring with loving around you that helps you make it.*[60]

One aspect of the loneliness that threatens a person comes as a result of fears of contagion. Other's responses to this fear also give the impression of abandonment. As one man expressed it: "One guy who was a close family friend would not shake my hand."[61] According to physicians, social workers, and patients, reactions such as this are common in cases of cancer and especially with AIDS. They leave the person alone and feeling abandoned.

In the study conducted by Bean et al., patients were asked what their knowledge of cancer had been before they were diagnosed. The typical response was that "cancer kills."[62] That is also the single most common association with AIDS. The identification of an illness with the prospect of death compounds the loneliness process by introducing the common difficulty that family and friends have in dealing with the impending death of a loved one.

In Bean's study, over one half of the patients who were asked to comment on their difficulties with family and friends expressed concerns about communication. Comments such as "Sometimes nobody feels like talking about it" and "Some people fall apart when you mention cancer"[63] express the typical experience of people who want to talk but have no one with whom they can talk. These comments suggest that a terminal illness is not a subject about which most people are willing to talk, even or perhaps especially when it involves someone with whom they share a close relationship. The patient therefore must adapt. This may be done by remaining silent or by choosing socially acceptable vocabulary. One person chose the word "tumor" rather than "cancer" when speaking to family and friends because it sounded better. In another instance, the mother of a young man with AIDS told people her son had leukemia for the same reason: socially, it was easier to say and hear.

When communication breaks down, loneliness is heightened as the person moves further and further away from others. It is unrealistic to expect a person to deal effectively with illness or death when those around him/her are denying, through their reluctance to speak of it, what is happening.

Because of its implications for care, it is worthwhile to look at the issue of abandonment in cases of AIDS a little more closely. Much of this does revolve around fear of contagion. Yet, given the fact that HIV is actually less infectious than such viruses as hepatitis B, it seems that there are other factors involved as well. Certainly one is that, once the virus is contracted, a person is considered to be infected for life. Also, if someone infected with HIV does develop AIDS, it is considered to be fatal. It is legitimate to ask if these facts interfere with good medical care.[64]

An incident at the University of Illinois Hospital in 1986 illustrates well the medical isolation that can occur in cases of AIDS. In this instance, a medical student refused to draw blood from a patient with AIDS. The student expressed concern about contracting the virus through accidental needlesticks. This refusal, and others like it, come in spite of evidence, that:

> ... *isolation procedures currently recommended for AIDS are adequate and that the risk of transmission within hospitals is low. Moreover, accidental needlestick exposure appears to provide little additional risk of HTLV-III transmission.*[65]

This attitude of reluctance to become clinically involved with a person with AIDS is not isolated to a few unfortunate instances. A 1987 survey found that, in general, nurses were concerned about the prospect of treating AIDS patients and those at high risk, at least for a prolonged time.[66] The survey showed that:

> *Two thirds reported family and friends had expressed concern about associating with hospital personnel who have contact with AIDS patients. There were even reports of spouses who were reluctant to allow his/her husband/wife to get too close to his/her own children.*

> *One third expressed concern about treating homosexually-oriented male patients or male prisoners who were patients because they belonged to high-risk groups for AIDS.*

50% said AIDS was likely to be transmitted through contact with an AIDS patient in spite of precautions.

51% were more afraid of treating a patient with AIDS than of treating a patient with infectious hepatitis.

7% would not hesitate to perform mouth-to-mouth resuscitation for a patient with AIDS, as compared with 9% who would not hesitate to do the same for someone with hepatitis.

48% believed HIV was likely to be transmitted through contact with clinical specimens in spite of precautions.

85% felt a nurse who was pregnant should not care for an AIDS patient.

39% stated they would have to request a transfer to another unit if they had to care for AIDS patients on a regular basis. This figure was 52% for those nurses who work in an intensive care unit (ICU).[67]

It is difficult to address the legitimate concerns of all those involved in healthcare and still offer good care. Whalen has suggested that the key issue in this discussion is the question of professionalism. By this, I understand him to mean the willingness of the healthcare provider to offer care that is knowledgeable of the risks, yet at the same time sensitive to the needs of the person who is ill. Refusing to perform what are considered to be routine and safe medical procedures or insisting on the use of protective garments when they are not warranted are just two examples that illustrate how concern for risks can mitigate care by introducing a note of isolation. Whalen's words concerning the role of students in healthcare make it clear that he views professionalism as a central aspect of the healthcare environment:

The real issue behind whether students should work with AIDS patients is whether students are professional enough to subject themselves to the unknown risks attendant on being a health care professional.[68]

All persons in the medical field take on risks. Some of these are well defined, whereas others are unknown. These risks must be acknowledged and respected. They cannot, however, be exaggerated. It is essential that people in healthcare not be selective about the scientific data given them concerning AIDS or any other disease. What is known, and not what is feared, needs to be the basis of care. Anything less will lead to the isolation and loneliness that the person most fears, particularly in the face of a terminal disease. The Health and Public Policy Committee of the American College of Physicians and the Council of the Infectious Diseases Society of America make this same point in a 1986 joint statement:

> *It is inappropriate for any health care employee to compromise treatment of patients with transmissible, lethal diseases such as AIDS on the grounds that such patients present unacceptable medical risks.*[69]

Self-Worth

As persons, everyone has various opinions of themselves. Some people think highly of themselves, whereas others think poorly. This opinion is drawn from both subjective and objective sources. Subjectively, it is drawn from the perception of who persons think they are and what they have to offer their community. Objectively, it is drawn from others' opinions of who the person is and what this person can offer. When these two opinions come together, there emerges a picture of one's self-worth, that is, the worth or value that a person places on his/her life and activity. At times, a person's self-worth may be threatened, and questions may arise as to the value of his/her personhood. This often happens through a process of depersonalization, the process by which a person's worth is devalued.

Anyone who has ever been in a hospital knows that depersonalization can begin, more through routine than intent, as soon as one walks into the admitting office and receives a wristband. If the medical staff is aware only of the person's illness, then the person as such, with all that personhood entails, is denied. This often happens when responsibility for the day-to-day decisions of the person are turned over to the medical team. A kind of stereotyping can also lead to this denial of personhood. This can occur when a person is ascribed as having certain characteristics that seem to belong to patients in general but are not necessarily appropriate to a particular person. For example, members of the staff may think of all patients as helpless and base care on that assumption. Treating everyone in this way ignores the desire of some, who may or may not be helpless, to preserve some independence.

Another form of stereotyping exists in instances when all people with AIDS are associated with homosexuality or drug abuse, or when all people with a homosexual orientation are seen as being carriers of HIV. In these instances, the person's full identity may be lost to his/her sexual identity or illness or to a presumed sexual identity.[70] At times, all anyone may be aware of is the physical fact of the disease or the person's real or presumed life style. When this happens, all care is directed toward a body, not a person.

Focusing only on the disease and stereotyping people into categories have one common feature: they both ignore the truth. The response of a young woman with leukemia expressed the frustration of being identified with a disease:

When you look at me, don't think of me as a patient or as a case of leukemia. Think of me as a person—as the person you knew before I became ill.[71]

It would be unfair to imply that it is only within the medical care profession that depersonalization takes place. It is also evident in American society as a whole, particularly in the work force. A five-year study funded by the California Division of the American Cancer Society illustrates this.[72] This study, conducted from 1980 to 1985 by Feldman, a professor of social work at the University of Southern California, examined the experiences of several hundred blue- and white-collar workers, all of whom were working at the time they were diagnosed as having cancer.

This study revealed that more than 50 percent of the white-collar workers and 84 percent of the blue-collar workers reported difficulties on the job that were directly related to the fact that they had cancer. These included demotions, being passed over for a promotion, or being forced to give up membership in the employer's group health insurance plan if they wanted to keep their jobs. Other psychological abuses included isolating and shunning the person on the one extreme and treating the person with excessive concern on the other.

Feldman also found that when people with cancer went to seek a job and their health histories became known, they suddenly became disqualified. Some reasons given for not hiring were that the job available would be too stressful, the person would miss too many days of employment, and the group insurance rate would rise.

The story of one man suffering from leukemia illustrates well the effects of stereotyping a person. Being seen only as an illness, he was robbed of the other qualities of his personal identity and was depersonalized by those around him.[73]

This young man had been hoping to go to medical school when he was first diagnosed with leukemia. After that, things began to change. After several months of treatment, he found that he had to withdraw his applications to several medical schools because he was too weak to take the National Board examinations. After the leukemia went into remission and he had regained much of his health, he was able to take the tests and passed

them. With prior knowledge of his illness, however, the schools found him
to be unacceptable:

> *Before I became sick, several schools had called me for interviews.
> But now, with cancer on my record, I was being dropped
> everywhere.*[74]

In addition to being rejected as a capable student because of an illness,
his life was subtly seen as being not worth the investment of time by
intimate others. When his engagement was announced, family and friends
"couldn't understand why any girl would get engaged to a guy who might
be dead in a year."[75]

With AIDS, this social prejudice has gone to an extreme. Thompson has
observed that many AIDS patients suffer from low self-esteem as a result:

> *Shattered self-esteem and recrimination from the public at large
> lessen the AIDS victim's opportunities to fight the disease or to find
> a significant experience in the process of dying of it.*[76]

Perhaps nowhere else is the issue of self-worth more critical than in the
cases of children with AIDS. Parents concerned about their own children
have repeatedly sought to keep children with AIDS out of public school
systems.[77] In November 1986, federal law was invoked in a case involving a
kindergarten student who had bitten another child. The district court ruled
that AIDS is a handicap protected under the Vocational Rehabilitation Act of
1973. The California school system was ordered to make a reasonable
attempt to accommodate the child.[78]

There have also been cases involving children who have ARC or family
members who have AIDS. In Orange County, CA, local parents sought to
prevent a child from attending school after testing positive for HIV.[79] In
Georgia, a six-year-old boy was prevented from attending school for three
months because his 11-month-old sister had become infected during
pregnancy by her mother and had died of AIDS. The child was admitted
after the NAACP threatened a lawsuit, but with the condition that the child
not live in the same house as his mother.[80] A lawsuit currently pending in
Florida involves seven-year-old Haitian triplets. Since being diagnosed with
ARC, the three boys have been taught a regular curriculum by a volunteer
teacher in an isolated setting. The children's father is suing to have them
admitted into a normal classroom setting.[81]

Some of the earliest discrimination disputes relating to AIDS have been
in the area of employment, and the number of job discrimination suits has
continued to grow. One of the first cases involved a young man who lost his
job in Florida because he had AIDS. The Florida courts ultimately held that

such a dismissal constituted discrimination against a handicapped person, which is unlawful under Florida law.[82] In August 1986, a lawsuit in Virginia resulted in a $20,000 settlement for a physician whose contract at a walk-in clinic was terminated when he was diagnosed with AIDS.[83] In Massachusetts, a suit by a telephone company employee with AIDS was settled out of court nearly one year after he was forced to leave his job. The company agreed to reinstate him in his former position.[84]

The legal question that has emerged is whether or not HIV infection, ARC, or AIDS constitutes a handicap. If they do, then people with these handicaps would be entitled to protection under the law. All 50 states have statutes that protect the handicapped, and at least 33 states have indicated that they will view AIDS and ARC as a handicap.[85] In these states, employers generally may not discharge, refuse to hire, or otherwise discriminate against such a person who is otherwise capable of performing the job. In some states, the protection of handicap discrimination laws has been extended to those who are merely perceived to have a handicap, regardless of whether or not they are actually impaired. Where this is the case, it is probable that people who have tested positive for HIV but who do not have any clinical symptoms of AIDS or ARC would also be protected.

The question of whether or not AIDS constitutes a true handicap was settled by a 1987 Supreme Court decision stating that people with AIDS are protected under section 504 of the Vocational Rehabilitation Act of 1973. This law provides limited protection to prohibit discrimination against federal employees, as well as those employees associated with federal programs, grants, and contracts. The law, which defines a handicapped person as one who has a physical or mental impairment that substantially limits one or more of the person's major life activities, applies to areas of employment, education, medical treatment, and other service or benefit areas.

In its seven to two decision, the Supreme Court rejected the arguments of the Justice Department that an employer's fears of contagion, whether reasonable or not, constituted a sufficient reason to relieve a person with a communicable disease from his/her job. The case heard by the court involved a Florida school teacher who had been dismissed because she had tuberculosis. The court ruled that employers receiving federal funds cannot deny jobs to people with contagious disease simply because of their own perceptions about the illness. The court went on to state:

It would be unfair to allow an employer to seize upon the distinction between the effects of the disease on others and the effects of a disease on a patient and use that distinction to justify discriminatory treatment.[86]

Other areas of discrimination that can lead to a loss of self-worth among people with AIDS has involved housing. In 1983, a New York physician's lease was terminated after it was learned that he treated people with AIDS. The court later determined that this was a violation of the New York Human Rights Law.[87] In the U.S. capital, objections were raised when plans were made to open a hospice for AIDS victims in a neighborhood in northeast Washington, DC. Homeowners feared that such a hospice in the neighborhood would lead to a lowering of property values. In California, a group of realtors has instituted a policy of informing prospective buyers when a former homeowner had AIDS.[88]

A group who is often forgotten but also suffers from the psychological effects of AIDS are those at risk of contracting the virus. Of particular concern are hemophiliac persons.

In spite of the assurances from the medical profession on the reliability of ELISA blood screening, concerns of receiving HIV-infected blood in a transfusion remain. A recent study of hemophiliac persons, their spouses, and their parents found a decrease in the average number of treatments per patient per month since the discovery of AIDS.[89] With respect to contagion, 59 percent of the hemophiliacs expressed concern about transmitting the disease to a spouse, and 57 percent of the spouses expressed concern about becoming infected. As a result, 21 percent of the hemophiliac persons and 10 percent of the spouses reported a decrease in sexual desires. Just less than 10 percent of the couples indicated that there had been a lessening of sexual activity in their relationship.

This study also brought out a communication difficulty that can exist between a hemophiliac person and a spouse. For example, although 57 percent of the spouses were concerned with HIV infection, only 37 percent of the hemophiliacs thought the spouse was concerned. Further, whereas almost 11 percent of the spouses sought to respond to this concern through a decrease in sexual activity, only 4.7 percent of the hemophiliacs thought that the spouse's sexual reluctance was related to the risk of infection. Such gaps in understanding between couples will almost certainly lead to questions concerning one's worth to another or oneself.

A conclusion of the study stated that, although the overall hemophiliac population is coping well with the risk of AIDS, some are at an increased risk for psychiatric morbidity, social isolation, hypochondriasis, and medical noncompliance.

This study dealt only with hemophilia, but the results do present the stresses and concerns likely to be present in other groups at risk for AIDS as well. This suggests that specific psychological intervention is often urgently needed to assist people with AIDS to maintain a positive sense of self-worth.

As would be expected, there has been an unprecedented demand by

AIDS patients and family members for psychological support. This need can be met partly through greater education on the part of the healthcare industry. The Patient Services Staff of AIDS Atlanta, a not-for-profit organization that provides services to AIDS patients and their families, has found that receiving healthcare from professionals who are very familiar with AIDS is of great importance to their clients.[90] Knowledgeable medical personnel are less likely to treat their patients in ways that increase the feelings of isolation and helplessness that often accompany AIDS and lead to a lower sense of personal worth. To date, AIDS Atlanta reports that 46 percent of its clients have requested assistance such as support groups for themselves and/or family, and 19 percent have requested individual counseling or therapy.[91] Still, Thompson reports that not enough is being done nationwide:

> *Even as we have established a firmer understanding of the nature of AIDS, we have not moved as rapidly as possible to deal with the psychologic effects of the disease on all parties of the illness.[92]*

DISEASE: COPING AND INTEGRATION

As can be seen, the impact of having a life-threatening disease and the treatment involved can be enormous for both the person and the family involved. The diagnosis brings about immediate thoughts of death, usually a lingering death. For the elderly person, the diagnosis often means one more life-threatening situation with which to deal. For the younger person, it can mean disaster and bring about profound changes in one's outlook on life.[93] The emotional response of the person to this situation is referred to as the process of *coping,* a term that "describes a continuum of attempts by the patients to maintain personal control over their lives."[94]

Coping is a process through which the person seeks to maintain self-esteem. This process may take the form of a positive effort in which the individual sustains normal activity or develops new activities to compensate and build esteem in new areas. In this way, the person seeks to increase control despite the illness, learns to care for him/herself, looks for self-improvement goals to overcome any disabilities, and attempts to actively seek information about the disease and the prognosis in order to participate in the decision-making process.

The process can also be a negative effort in which the person develops behavioral patterns that can ultimately injure self-esteem. In this instance, the person may deny the seriousness of the disease, delegate all decision making to others, regress into childlike behavior to obtain emotional support, or act out violently to punish others for their "luck" at being healthy. Douglas and Druss suggest that some patients will use an illness to escape from the responsibilities of everyday life. They also state that, in some instances, the person's bodily disfigurement will actually reflect his/her internalized perception of a defective self-worth.[95]

There are many different aspects involved in the coping process, a typical one being the initiation of defense mechanisms. These serve the important purpose of protecting the person from overwhelming fears, especially the fears often associated with dying. These defenses regulate the type and amount of information that the person is likely to seek and receive. Defense mechanisms will be discussed in greater depth in Chapter Three. It is primarily by way of introduction that they are presented here.

Defense mechanisms are, to a large extent, unconsciously and automatically initiated for the purpose of managing anxiety, impulses, hostility, resentments, and frustrations. This is accomplished through the emotions of denial, projection, distortion, rejection, rationalization, reaction formation, and sublimation. These emotional defenses are a crucial aspect of the person's day-to-day life and can be viewed as being equally as important as the body's physiological defenses of the immune system.[96] A certain amount of adaptive denial may be necessary to keep one from becoming morbid in the face of constant emotional contact with a serious situation.

Emotional defenses are vital not only during the initial shock of the diagnosis, but also later during the period of treatment or the time leading up to death. As a result of the stress of the disease and the treatment involved, the person often finds his/her ability to handle the events of a daily routine diminished. In these instances, the person may rely on emotional defenses to deal not only with the disease, but also with the events in everyday life. For example, denial serves not only to shield the person from being overwhelmed by the diagnosis, but later also protects the person from being overwhelmed by the changes in life style necessitated by the illness and treatment.

Much has already been said concerning the stress involved with cancer and AIDS. One clinical example will give some insight into the stress of treatment. In reference to her chemotherapy treatments, one woman recalled in an interview:

> *It made me very, very sick. I used to go for treatments on Monday, and every week it was hell ... I had times when I was spitting blood and sometimes the medicine was so strong my mind would kind of—I don't know—hallucinate. I really had to fight to hold on.*[97]

Tuesday would also be a difficult day, but by Wednesday she would be fine. When Sunday evening came, however, she would begin to experience fear and nausea, knowing that she had to go in the next day for another treatment. In the winter, she would pray for snow so that it would be impossible to drive into town. Of the waiting room before treatment, she said:

> *After a while, you have to psych yourself up to walk in there because it's really—this is just plain old corny—but it's like you're living in hell. You see them turning yellow, then disappearing, and it's like you're living in two worlds. . . . This one, where people are in hell, is the real one. The other one, your family, your children out there . . . it's a fantasy, far away, not real.*[98]

It is clear that, for the person in therapy, such common experiences as being cut off in traffic or the noise of a door slamming often provoke a more extreme reaction than they would under normal circumstances.

Defenses are meant to protect the person from the frightening feelings of annihilation that accompany the diagnosis and difficult treatment of illness. This is sometimes accomplished through *entitlement* and is common among many patients. In this context, entitlement refers to the belief on the person's part that since he/she has been deprived or injured in one area of life, he/she deserves some compensation in some other areas. Entitlement helps the person to maintain self-worth by seeing him/herself as "worthy" of some privileges even as the body is growing progressively weaker. This quest for special treatment is sometimes shown in the asking of multiple and lengthy questions. Although questioning is important and healthy, when the process is extended for the purpose of gaining attention, it is probably a case of entitlement. When this is the case, the person's value and worth should be clearly demonstrated by others to alleviate fears of rejection and the need to seek out affirmation.

Depression is another common and appropriate emotional response. With people who suffer from depression, it is important for the medical team to learn if there has been any previous history of depression and to what extent this depression impairs functioning. Depression is often accompanied by weight loss, sleep disturbance, and anorexia. These symptoms often accompany cancer and AIDS as well. When they appear, it is first necessary to determine whether or not such symptoms are the result of the disease or are part of an emotional response to the disease, that is, whether they are of physical or psychological origin. If it seems that they are not related directly to the disease itself, some type of psychiatric intervention is usually called for, even in instances where the depression itself is considered to be appropriate. Concerning the possibility of depression, it has been observed that people who have maintained successful coping strategies while healthy are often more able to mobilize compensating interpersonal achievement and identification activities when ill. This ability can assume greater importance as death approaches.[99]

It is not known with any certainty to what extent coping mechanisms directly affect a person's ability to recover health, yet the work of Simonton et al. and others cited earlier indicate that such a correlation is not to be ignored completely. In general, it can be said that, no matter what role the ability to cope plays in maintaining or recovering physical health, it is evident that coping, particularly through defense mechanisms, is an important way for the person to pursue the human task and to achieve and maintain well-being in the face of illness or death. Well-being can be restored and maintained through coping that defends and protects the integrity of the person. This facilitates the process of integration by allowing for some control within the present situation. This, in turn, allows the person to pursue the human task and place or discover some order and meaning in the illness or the dying so that it can be lived out.

To sum up, therefore, when a person becomes ill and his/her integrity is threatened in whatever way, the person has a natural and innate need and ability to recover well-being. The person may not regain health but can strive to return to a sense of integration and wholeness by finding meaning within his/her situation. This is accomplished, at least in part, through coping. In this way, the person moves toward becoming once again an integrated and well person. As one person phrased it:

> *It's incredible how much you can lose, how disfigured you can become, but still laugh, still hold onto life. So you cope because you know there are worse things in life than losing an arm or a leg.*[100]

NOTES

1. Elida A. Evan, *A Psychological Study of Cancer,* Dodd, Mead & Co., New York, 1926.
2. Lawrence L. LeShan, *You Can Fight for Your Life: Emotional Factors in the Causation of Cancer,* M. Evans & Co., New York, 1977.
3. See, for example, Leon Jaroff, "Can Attitude Affect Cancer?" *Time,* June 24, 1985, p. 69.
4. Peggy Boyd, *The Silent Wound: A Startling Report on Breast Cancer and Sexuality,* Addison-Wesley, Reading, MA, 1984. Boyd suggests that unresolved adolescent conflicts about sexuality inflict a silent wound that, in later life, can increase a woman's susceptibility to disease, including breast cancer. See also Norman Cousins, *Anatomy of an Illness as Perceived by the Patient: Reflections*

on Healing and Regeneration, Bantam Books, New York, 1979. Cousins tells how he cured himself of spinal arthritis by adopting a healthy mental attitude, watching comedy movies to induce laughter, and taking large doses of Vitamin C. See also Andrew Weil, *Health and Healing: Understanding Conventional and Alternative Medicine,* Houghton Mifflin, Boston, 1983, pp. 56-57. Weil speaks of nine principles of health and illness, the fifth being that all illness is psychosomatic because as persons we are mind-bodies; thus what affects the mind affects the body.

5. Barrie R. Cassileth et al., "Psychological Correlates of Survival in Advanced Malignant Disease?" *The New England Journal of Medicine* 312, 1985, pp. 1551-1555. Although admitting that psychological factors may play a role in causing or influencing the course of malignant disease, Cassileth sees this as only one link in a very long causal chain. This study of patients with advanced, high-risk malignant diseases suggests that the inherent biology of the disease alone determines the prognosis, overriding the potentially mitigating influence of psychosocial factors. See also Marcia Angell, "Disease as a Reflection of the Psyche," *The New England Journal of Medicine* 312, 1985, pp. 1570-1572. In this editorial, Angell argues that although people are responsible for their own health, the belief that disease is a direct reflection of one's mental state is largely folklore.

6. R.L. Carter, "Pathological Aspects," in *The Management of Terminal Disease,* ed. Cicely M. Saunders, Edward Arnold Publishers Ltd., London, 1978, p. 29.

7. Robert C. Gallo, "The AIDS Virus," *Science* 256, 1987, pp. 46-56.

8. National Center for Health Statistics report in "AIDS Myths," *Newsweek,* Nov. 16, 1987, p. 6.

9. J.W. Smith, "HIV transmitted by intercourse but not by kissing" (letter), *British Medical Journal* 294, 1987, pp. 446-447.

10. Margaret C. Fisher, "Transfusion-Associated Acquired Immunodeficiency Syndrome—What is the Risk?" *Pediatrics* 79, 1987, pp. 157-160.

11. Fisher, p. 158.

12. Delsworth G. Harnkish et al., "Early Detection of HIV Infection in a Newborn" (correspondence), *The New England Journal of Medicine* 316, 1987, pp. 272-273.

13. "AIDS-Infection Rates High Among Pregnant in City," Associated Press, *The Washington Post,* Nov. 20, 1987, p. A16.

14. "CDC Update: Acquired Immunodeficiency Syndrome—United States," *Morbidity and Mortality Weekly Report* 35, 1986, pp. 17-21. See also Stephen David Barbour, "Acquired Immunodeficiency Syndrome of Childhood," *Pediatric Clinics of North America* 34, 1987, pp. 247-268.

15. C. Everett Koop, *Surgeon General's Report on Acquired Immune Deficiency Syndrome,* reprinted in *Journal of the American Medical Association* 256, 1986, pp. 2764-2789.

16. Margaret W. Hilgartner, "AIDS and Hemophilia" (editorial), *The New England Journal of Medicine* 317, 1987, pp. 18-19.

17. Koop, pp. 2764-2789.

18. For a complete list of the criteria that constitute a diagnosis of AIDS, see "Revision of the CDC Surveillance Case Definition for Acquired Immunodeficiency Syndrome," *Morbidity and Mortality Weekly Report* 36, 1987, pp. 3s-15s.
19. Carmelita U. Tuazon and Ann M. Labriola, "Management of Infectious and Immunological Complications of Acquired Immunodeficiency Syndrome (AIDS): Current and Future Prospects," *Drugs* 33, 1987, pp. 66-84.
20. Harry Hollander, "Practical Management of Common AIDS Related Medical Problems," *Western Journal of Medicine* 237, 1987, pp. 146, 237-240.
21. D.I. Abrams et al., "Persistent Diffuse Lymphadenopathy in Homosexual: Endpoint or Prodrome," *Annuals of Internal Medicine* 100, 1984, pp. 801-808.
22. See, for example, D.M. Barnes, "Brain Damage by AIDS Under Active Study" (news), *Science* 235, 1987, pp. 1574-1577; and C.H. Beresford, "Dementia in Human Immunodeficiency Virus Infection" (letter), *New Zealand Medical Journal* 100, 1987, p. 32.
23. John A. Roberts, *The Rights of the Critically Ill,* Bantam Books, New York, 1985, p. 164.
24. These categories are taken from Christopher C. Gates, "Psychological Issues in Cancer," in *Cancer: A Manual for Practitioners,* 5th ed., ed. Blake Cady, American Cancer Society, Boston, 1978, pp. 80-90 (hence referred to as *Cancer: A Manual*). See also Melvin J. Krant, "What Cancer Means to Society," *Proceedings of the American Cancer Society Third National Conference on Human Values and Cancer,* American Cancer Society, Washington, DC, 1981, pp. 15-19 (hence referred to as *Proceedings/Human Values and Cancer*).
25. Roberts, p. 80.
26. Anne Munley, *The Hospice Alternative: A New Concept for Death and Dying,* Basic Books, New York, 1983, p. 110.
27. Anselm L. Strauss, *Chronic Illness and the Quality of Life,* The C.V. Mosby Co., St. Louis, 1984, p. 9.
28. Roberts, p. 78.
29. Curtis B. Pepper, "The Visitors: Patients Who Conquered Cancer," *New York Times Magazine,* Jan. 29, 1984, p. 17.
30. Roberts, p. 79.
31. Madeleine Corbeil, "Nursing Process for a Patient with a Body Image Disturbance," *Nursing Clinics of North America* 6, 1971, pp. 156-157.
32. Robert L. Frierson and Steven B. Lippmann, "Psychologic Implications of AIDS," *American Family Physician* 35, 1987, p. 113.
33. Robert L. Blaney and Gary F. Piccola, "Psychological Issues Related to AIDS," *Journal of the Medical Association of Georgia* 76, 1987, p. 29.
34. Pepper, p. 26.
35. Roberts, p. 80.
36. Pepper, p. 20.
37. See, for example, Phyllis B. Taylor, "Understanding Sexuality in the Dying Patient," *Nursing '83* 13, 1983, pp. 54-55.
38. Frierson and Lippmann, p. 112.
39. Blaney and Piccola, p. 30.
40. Munley, p. 117.

41. Pepper, p. 28.
42. Laurie Bobskill, "Clergyman Dying of AIDS Ministers to Others (an Interview)," *Sunday Republican* 9, Nov. 8, 1987, p. 81.
43. Glynis Bean et al., "Coping Mechanisms of Cancer Patients: A Study of 33 Patients Receiving Chemotherapy," *CA—A Cancer Journal for Clinicians* 30, 1980, pp. 256-259. See also William J. Worden, "Teaching Adaptive Coping to Cancer Patients," *Proceedings/Human Values and Cancer,* pp. 129-138.
44. Bean, p. 257.
45. Bean, p. 257.
46. See, for example, Leonard R. Derogatis, Martin D. Abeloff, and Nick Melisaratos, "Psychological Coping Mechanisms and Survival Time in Metastatic Breast Cancer," *Journal of the American Medical Association* 242, 1979, pp. 1504-1508.
47. Frierson and Lippmann, p. 113.
48. David Agle, Henry Gluck, and Glenn F. Pierce, "The Risk of AIDS: Psychologic Impact on the Hemophiliac Population," *General Hospital Psychiatry* 9, 1987, pp. 11-17.
49. Frierson and Lippmann, p. 113.
50. Roberts, pp. 291-292.
51. J. Bradley Hoskisson, *Loneliness: An Explanation, A Cure,* Citadel Press, New York, 1965, p. 26.
52. Hoskisson, p. 36.
53. Roberts, pp. 142-144.
54. Los Angeles County–University of Southern California Cancer Center, *Psychological Aspects of Cancer,* LAC–USC Publication, Los Angeles, 1983, p. 3.
55. J. Englebert Dunphy, "Annual Discourse: On Caring for the Patient with Cancer," in *Cancer: A Manual,* p. 343.
56. Bean et al., p. 258.
57. O. Carl Simonton, Stephanie Matthews-Simonton, and James L. Creighton, *Getting Well Again: A Step-by-Step Self-Help Guide to Overcoming Cancer for Patients and Their Families,* Bantam Books, New York, 1978, pp. 87-88.
58. Blaney and Piccola, p. 32.
59. Pepper, p. 18. See also W.P. Laird Myers, "Attitudes of Physicians as Revealed in their Approaches to Patients with Advanced Cancer," in *Proceedings/Human Values and Cancer,* pp. 59-68.
60. Pepper, p. 18.
61. Rick Taylor, "Cancer Patients Face Prejudice on Job," *Springfield* (MA) *Sunday Republican,* Nov. 25, 1984, sec. II, p. B1.
62. Bean et al., p. 257.
63. Bean et al., p. 258.
64. Marylou Webster, "Are A.I.D.S. Patients Getting Good Nursing Care?" *Nursing Life,* 1987, pp. 48-53.
65. Martin S. Hirsch et al., "Risk of Nosocomial Infection with Human T-Cell Lymphotropic Virus III (HTLV-III)," *The New England Journal of Medicine* 312, 1985, p. 3; Gary P. Wormer et al., "Needlestick Injuries During the Care of Patients with AIDS," *The New England Journal of Medicine* 310, 1984, p. 1461;

and "Acquired Immune Deficiency Syndrome (AIDS) and Precautions for Clinical and Laboratory Staffs," *Mortality and Morbidity Weekly Report* 31, 1982, pp. 560-570, 32, 1983, pp. 450-451.

66. Michael Blumenfield, Peggy Jordano Smith, and Jane Milazzo, "Survey of Attitudes of Nurses Working with AIDS Paients," *General Hospital Psychiatry* 9, 1987, pp. 58-63.

67. Blumenfield et al., pp. 58-63.

68. James P. Whalen, "Participation of Medical Students in the Care of Patients with AIDS," *Journal of Medical Education* 62, 1987, pp. 53-54.

69. "Acquired Immunodeficiency Syndrome," *Annals of Internal Medicine* 104, 1986, pp. 575-581.

70. The Roman Catholic Church speaks of this need to avoid stereotyping with respect to homosexuality when it states: "Today, the Church provides a badly needed context for the care of the person when she refuses to consider the person as 'heterosexual' or 'homosexual' and insists that every person has a fundamental identity." Congregation for the Doctrine of the Faith, "Letter to Bishops of the Catholic Church on the Pastoral Care of Homosexual Persons," *L'Observatore Romano* 45, Nov. 10, 1986, p. 3.

71. LAC–USC, p. 14.

72. Taylor, p. B1.

73. Pepper, pp. 24-28.

74. Pepper, p. 28.

75. Pepper, p. 26.

76. Leslie M. Thompson, "Dealing with AIDS and Fear: Would You Accept Cookies From an AIDS Patient?" *Southern Medical Journal* 80, 1987, p. 231.

77. For an excellent overview of cases involving discrimination against persons with AIDS, see Gene W. Matthews and Verla S. Neslund, "The Initial Impact of AIDS on Public Health Law in the United States—1986," *Journal of the American Medical Association* 257, 1987, pp. 344-352; and James H. Coil, III, "Legal Issues Involving Aids," *Journal of the Medical Association of Georgia* 76, 1987, pp. 64-68.

78. See *Thomas v. Atascadero Unified School District,* No. 886-609AHS(BY) C.D. Cal. Nov. 17, 1986.

79. See *Phipps v. Saddleback Unified School District,* No. 474981 (Orange County Super. Ct., Feb. 18, 1986).

80. Matthews et al., p. 345.

81. See *C.C. v. Dade County School Board,* No. 86-1513-CIV (S.D. Florida, filed July 18, 1986).

82. See *Shuttleworth v. Broward County,* No. 85-6623-CIV (S.D. Florida, filed July 18, 1986).

83. See *John Doe v. Primary Care Corp.,* C.A. No. 86-377-A (E.D. Va. 1986).

84. See *Cronen v. New England Telephone & Telegraph Co.,* No. 80332 (Suffolk County, MA, Super. Ct., settled Oct. 16, 1986).

85. Coil, p. 65.

86. Nancy Henderson, "Supreme Court reverses AIDS judgment," *Nature* 326, March 1987, p. 115.

87. See No. 43604/83 (N.Y. Sup. Ct., Dec. 20, 1983).
88. Matthews et al., p. 349.
89. Agle et al., pp. 11-17.
90. Sarah W. Holmes and Jesse Peel, "Meeting the Mental Health Challenge of AIDS and Related Disorders," *Journal of the Medical Association of Georgia* 76, Jan. 1987, pp. 33-43.
91. Holmes and Peel, p. 34.
92. Thompson, p. 230.
93. See, for example, Victor and Rosemary Zorza, *A Way to Die,* Alfred A. Knopf, New York, 1980; Paul Tsongas, *Heading Home,* Alfred A. Knopf, New York, 1984; and U.S. Dept. of Health and Human Services, "Cancer in the Adult," "Cancer in the Young," in *Coping with Cancer: A Resource for the Health Professional,* DHHS, National Cancer Institute, Bethesda, MD, NIH Publication no. 80-2080, Sept. 1980, pp. 7-46, 47-78.
94. Bean et al., p. 256.
95. Carolyn T. Douglas and Richard G. Druss, "Denial of Illness: A Reappraisal," *General Hospital Psychiatry* 9, 1987, pp. 53-57.
96. Gates, p. 82.
97. Pepper, p. 16.
98. Pepper, p. 16.
99. Gates, p. 85.
100. Pepper, p. 16.

3 The Dying Person: The Possibility of Reconciliation with Death

This chapter will examine the person as one who is dying. As in the previous chapter on health and sickness, the approach will be to look at dying and death as it threatens the integrity of the person.

It is beyond the scope of this book to present a detailed and exact analysis of death itself. That is properly the work of thanatology. Although some reference will be made to the notion of death per se, particularly in reference to historical and contemporary attitudes, the emphasis of this chapter will be to illustrate the act of dying as a subjective, personal experience.[1] This presentation will rely principally on the works of Kübler-Ross and her five stages of death.[2]

Finally, a critique of contemporary society's attitudes toward death will be given. The chapter will conclude by showing that, although humanity's attempts at reconciliation may fail, a personal acceptance of one's own death is possible.

ATTITUDES TOWARD DEATH

Historical Attempts to be Reconciled with Death

Dying is an integral part of life, as natural and predictable as being born. Whereas birth is considered to be an occasion for celebration, however, death has become taboo, a dreaded and sometimes unspeakable issue, one that is to be avoided by every means possible. Perhaps this is because death is a reminder of human vulnerability in spite of technological advances in medicine. Death can be delayed but not escaped entirely. People, no less than any other creature, are destined to die. Furthermore, death is indiscriminate: everyone must die, whether rich or poor, famous or unknown, good or evil.

All the people on this earth will die; most, if not all, at any given moment, will fear it. At least some of this fear may be rooted in death's universality, especially among those who strive to control their own existence. Ariès speaks of humanity's need to control death in much the same way as humanity has sought to control sexual activity.[3] Insofar as we can determine the time, place, and manner of death, we can, at least minimally, be reconciled with our mortality.

Historically, many attempts have been made to somehow bring about this reconciliation.[4] These include the following six areas.

Hedonism. Perhaps the most obvious attempt to deal with death is found in the "eat, drink, and be merry for tomorrow we die" attitude of hedonism. Such an attitude is basically fatalistic and seeks to get all that life can offer before it is too late.

Pessimism. The opposite of hedonism, pessimism concludes that life is wretched and that death is a preferred evil. Pessimism gives way to an attitude of resignation in the face of death, the experience of merely giving up. As such, it stands in sharp contrast to the acceptance of death that will be discussed later in this chapter.

One indicator of an attitude of pessimism within a society is the incidence of suicide. In a society in which life is rated at so low a value that death is held to be the lesser evil, suicide may emerge as a basic human right, and its practice will be considered respectable and in some cases meritorious or even obligatory.

Other indicators may include euthanasia, some instances of abortion, as well as some decisions that dictate who should be kept alive, who should receive treatment, and so forth. When life is seen as being of little positive value, there are few good reasons to maintain or assist a life that involves suffering, hardships, or handicaps.

Circumvention of Death Through Some Physical Countermeasures. Practiced in the extreme in ancient Egypt with the mummifications of the Pharaohs, this notion is based on the premise that the deceased person's life can be somehow prolonged after death if the corpse is preserved. Provisions may be made to provide, food, drink, and various other services that the person enjoyed during earthly life.

Circumvention by Living on in Those Who Remain. Historically, many communities and individuals have attempted to leave a legacy behind in testimony of their existence. This can be seen in the Book of Genesis and the promise made to Abraham. This was not a promise that he would enjoy eternal life but that his descendants would be as numerous as the sand on the seashore (Gn 12:2; 17:4; 18:18; 22:17). Toynbee suggests that, regardless of whether or not the prospect of becoming the Father of the Hebrew peoples reconciled Abraham to the prospect of his own death, it is evident that the promises made to Abraham by Yahweh were held, at least by the authors and editors of the Book of Genesis, to be more valuable and more satisfying than any promise of personal immortality.[5]

Today, individuals often try to circumvent the effects of death by leaving behind a legacy to perpetuate their memory. This legacy usually takes the form of wealth, power, or fame. In this, the hope is founded that one can live on in the life and memory of succeeding generations.

Self-Liberation from Self-Centeredness by Merging Oneself in Ultimate Reality. In this approach, the person seeks to be merged into oneness with all that is real in order to be free from all that is unreal. It is a notion found primarily in Eastern thought, particularly among Buddhists.

This philosophy holds that the goal of life is to merge oneself into all of reality, becoming one with existence itself. This is accomplished through the freeing of the self from any sense of desire. Once one has obtained this state of "nirvana," the person lives on in oneness with all that is for all eternity. In such a philosophy, death is not the primary difficulty with which the person must be reconciled, for the person will keep returning after death in a series of incarnations until this state of nirvana is attained. What the person will need to become reconciled with is that cycle of rebirths.

Belief in the Resurrection of the Human Body. This idea has often been associated with a last and general judgment of the dead in Christianity, Islam, and Zoroastrianism. In Pharisaic Judaism, this resurrection was a privilege extended only to those found worthy.

Tied closely to a belief in a resurrection is the hope of a heaven and the fear of a hell. This belief attempts to deal with death by influencing its outcome. Through a belief in reward and punishment, a person is able to direct personal conduct and attitudes to determine the state of life after death. Although death itself cannot be avoided, at least its "victory" and "sting" can be taken away by those who have some control over the consequences of death in a life to come. (Cor 1:15, 50-57).

Contemporary Views on Dying

The approach in dealing with death in today's society appears to be simply avoid the problem altogether. May uses the parable of the Good Samaritan to illustrate society's "passing by the other side" and concludes:

A striking feature of our management of the problem of old age, illness, and mental disturbance is our segregation of the populations so afflicted from the society at large.[6]

The same can be said of those who are dying, making the subject of death, in the words of Gorer, "pornographic":

In the twentieth century ... there seems to have been an unremarked shift in prudery; whereas copulation has become more and more "mentionable," particularly in the Anglo-Saxon societies, death has become more and more "unmentionable"as a natural process.[7]

This perception of death can be explained, at least in part, by the emergence in the United States of the hospital over the home as the primary place of care and death. This has had the effect of moving the death scene out of the public view. Today people die less visibly. The result is that what used to be a very real experience in everyone's life has become a vague abstraction about which people read. Even in this, there is some disinterest because it so difficult, if not impossible, to see death in regard to oneself.

In the past, family members often washed, dressed, and otherwise prepared the corpse in anticipation of mourning and burial. Today, people generally leave this to the mortician. The result has been that a great number of people today have never even seen a dead body. Nisbet makes the following observation:

Inevitably, cremation and instant dispatch of the ashes crowd out burial. Nor can it be claimed that this behavior is mute recognition of the disappearance of available land for cemeteries, for people at other times thought nothing of using and reusing graves, and there were charnel houses for the bones.[8]

When people do confront death, it is most often in the form of a beautified corpse, which sometimes does not even resemble the deceased. This practice seems to be an attempt to avoid death's impact by allowing people to find solace in how "good" or "peaceful" the person looks. A person is not said to have "died," but rather to have "passed on" or been "called for." It is rare that the reality of death is expressed so clearly as in the words of one gentleman who, when asked at a funeral parlor how he thought the deceased looked, responded with a simple, accurate, and unexpected "She looks dead."

This contemporary movement away from death, which seems to be rooted as well in primordial images of death in folklore literature, dream life, and ritual behavior that speak of death in symbols of "hiding,"[9] has given rise to many popular conceptions concerning the reality of death and the people who are dying. Some of these conceptions are:[10]

1. Only suicidal and psychotic people are willing to die. Even when death is inevitable, no one wants to die.
2. Fear of death is the most natural and basic fear of all human beings. The closer one comes to death, the greater the intensity of this fear.[11]
3. Reconciliation with and preparation for death are impossible to achieve. Therefore, when one is with a dying person, the best course of action is to say as little as possible, avoid all questions concerning death, and use whatever means necessary to deny, dissimulate, and avoid open confrontation.
4. People who are dying do not really want to know they are dying. If they did, they would ask more questions. To force a discussion or to insist on unwelcome information is risky, since the patient may give up all hope. This could lead to a deep depression, the hastening of death, or even suicide.
5. After speaking with family members, the physician should treat the dying person as long as possible. When further assistance appears to be fruitless, the person should be left alone except for the relief of pain. He/she will then withdraw and die in peace without further disturbance or anguish.
6. It is reckless, if not cruel, to inflict unnecessary suffering on the person dying or the family. The person is doomed anyway, so nothing can really make any difference. Survivors should accept the futility of the situation and realize that they will, in time, get over the loss.
7. Physicians, in view of their scientific training and clinical experience, can deal with all phases of the dying process. Any consultation with psychiatrists or social workers is unnecessary because the emotional and psychological sides of dying are vastly overemphasized. The clergy might be called on in this situation, but only because death is imminent. After death occurs, the medical team has no further obligation toward that person or the family.

Whether or not these popular conceptions are correct is not important at the moment. What is important is the central insight they share: death is foreign to the subjective, personal experience and to be avoided at all costs. This can be accomplished by keeping dying people alive, abandoning someone when death is inevitable so that one need not face another's failure, or by refusing to deal with the grief associated with death by somehow rising above the situation and being brave and strong.

These conceptions indicate that today's society does not see death as part of human existence. Death has become unfamiliar. People find it difficult to conceive of death as being natural, as when one goes to bed and simply does not wake up the next morning. Instead, when people do have to conceive of death, they often see it as something malignant and catastrophic, a destructive intervention from the outside that hits people suddenly and unprepared.

What can be seen in the historical and contemporary attempts of humanity to be reconciled with death is no reconciliation at all. Reconciliation involves a coming to terms with something. Here there is only an avoidance, a denial of death as a subjective, personal experience. Each of these attempts merely seeks to get around death, to somehow find a way to not really die. In this attempt, they fail.

In reality, it appears that humanity has not sought to be reconciled with death but has sought instead to establish justifications for not being involved in death. In so doing, humanity does not confront dying or death for what it is and how it is done. The personal experience of death is lost, as are the insights into how the dying might be cared for and how the suffering of the dying might be eased so that they may die well. To gain these insights, it is necessary to look not at how humanity has sought to get around the notion of death, but at the subjective, personal experience of how persons actually die.

DYING: THE SUBJECTIVE, PERSONAL EXPERIENCE

Facing Death

The diagnosis of a life-threatening illness has the impact of shattering the orderly and predictable unfolding of time. Suddenly, life plans and aspirations become indefinite. The person does not know how long he/she has to live, nor does the person know how the end will come. Suddenly everything is contingent. Munley quotes one patient describing it this way:

> *The worst thing is not knowing when. I know that it's going to happen, but I don't know when and I don't like this. There is no control. No way of being able to say I have this amount of time and then I'll die.*[12]

Sourkes notes that the kind of stress and the degree to which this stress affects the individual, as well as the family and the hospital staff, will depend on what point the patient has reached in one's "life cycle," that cycle of life that begins with birth and proceeds through a period of growing up into old age.[13]

For one who is elderly, this diagnosis may bring about anxieties of one more disability added to the others generally associated with getting old. The diagnosis may heighten fears of isolation and abandonment. On the other hand, it may come with a sense of inevitability, particularly if the person can look back on a long and fulfilled life. For many, there may be the satisfaction of completion that could soften the impact of the diagnosis. Others, whose lives have been a constant struggle, may feel overwhelmed at the thought that life has dealt one final tragedy.

For someone who is a young or middle-aged adult, there will be a greater sense of life being cut short. Just as goals and aspirations come into a clearer focus, the horizon becomes sharply delimited. People often express a sense of being cheated. Just when goals begin to become possible, they suddenly become impossible. This realization has a far greater impact on the person than the realization that some goals simply will not be attained, as with the coming of middle age. For the young person who is diagnosed as being terminally ill, all goals fade into oblivion. In the words of one person: "You feel as if you have been chopped in half. You can only make tentative gestures."

In the instance of a child or an adolescent, the effect of a diagnosis of a terminal illness does more than cut one's life short. It also introduces chaos into the assumed sequence of life, the sequence that has parents dying before their children:

> *A time of role reversal is expected, when children will care for dying parents. When parents instead find themselves watching their child face death, a sense of tragic absurdity prevails. Not only is time shortened, but its order is shattered.*[14]

This disruption of the natural order has a profound effect on parents because it is often perceived as a betrayal of trust. People trust that life is going to unfold in a particular way, that nature is going to work according to a particular set of rules. The death of a child breaks all those rules. This betrayal of the person by nature can introduce into the parents' lives a deeply rooted sense of insecurity. If nature cannot be trusted, then who or what can be? The death of a child often has the effect of calling into question many of those relationships upon which the person has come to depend to deal with different life crises.

There can be little preparation for the separation resulting from the death of a child because there has been no psychological preparation, such as occurs when children grow up and begin to move toward their own life ambitions. The impending death of an adolescent who is just beginning to move toward the exercise of some degree of independence is difficult to face as that movement is disrupted, halted, or reversed. The grief associated

with the death of a child often emerges as well from the realization that he/
she has not had the time to even begin to form any life dreams.

Parkes describes the time when one is faced with a diagnosis of a
terminal illness as a period in which one's basic life assumptions are
challenged.[15] Regardless of the point at which one finds oneself in the life
cycle, the news that one will not progress further demands that past
assumptions give way. Ideally, new assumptions that match the new reality
will be formulated.

This realization that life goals must change to fit a new reality follows
much the same pattern as the realization process that follows any major life
change or loss. There is grief in any situation in which a person is forced, by
changing circumstances, to give up one view of the world and accept
another, especially one for which he/she is not prepared. The person moves
from a state of incomprehension and numbness to a period of intense, inner
struggle in which an awareness of change conflicts with a strong impulse to
keep things the way they are. In the case of another's death, a need arises to
somehow recover the person or the relationship that has been lost. This is
generally followed by a phase of dejection and hopelessness in which the
person becomes increasingly aware of the discrepancy between his/her
vision of the world with all its hopes and dreams and the limited world that
now exists.

Finally, the person slowly begins to establish a new set of assumptions
to replace those that have become irrelevant. In a sense, people who find
themselves or those close to them about to die need to discover a new
identity. The wife begins to think of herself as a widow, the man who has a
disabling illness stops thinking of himself as a provider, and the one who is
dying begins to prepare to die.

This transition is not necessarily a smooth one. People tend to shift back
and forth from old assumptions to new, still tentative ones. However, most
people who have suffered a major loss do eventually experience a regaining
of strength. They use words such as "recovery," as if they had been through
some kind of sickness, and "reintegration" or "acceptance" to describe the
stability found in coming to terms with their new reality. Once the transition
has been made, life can go on.

Five "Stages" of Dying

In order to understand how a person might achieve this reintegration,
acceptance, or to use my own terminology, "well-being" in dying, it will be
helpful to take a closer look at the experience of dying and the way people
live out this time of transition. In this I will refer to the works of
Kübler-Ross.[16]

The ideas of Kübler-Ross have come under a good deal of criticism in recent years, particularly over her use of the expression "stages" when speaking of the dying process.[17] It is for this reason that the expression is in quotations. The word itself is misleading, perhaps even a misnomer. However, even in the work of those who criticize her, there is validation and confirmation of the personal experience that she is describing. For this reason, I choose to use her works and "stages" as the foundation for this chapter, although not without some caution.

My first caution has already been stated: "stages" is a difficult term. The expression implies a logical and consecutive development, suggesting that it is conceivable that there is a right and a wrong way to die. This is not the case. Shneidman writes that, in reality, there is a wide range of human emotions, few in some and dozens in others, that are experienced in a variety of orderings, reorderings, and arrangements.[18] Kübler-Ross admits this herself when she writes:

I hope that I am making it clear that patients do not necessarily follow a classical pattern from the stage of denial to the stage of anger, to bargaining, to depression, and acceptance.[19]

Part of this difficulty is found in the fact that the nature of a terminal disease is itself irregular and unpredictable. The person does not simply die, but rather experiences many little deaths in that experience. The examples presented in Chapter Two of how the integrity of the person is threatened by disease, as well as Parkes' comments on dying as a time of transition, give a clear indication that the person will experience many instances of different and sometimes conflicting emotions, even simultaneously.

Nevertheless, the stages to which Kübler-Ross refers are valid and valuable in an understanding of the experience of dying. They describe the overall coping mechanism that the person calls into service in the process of regaining wholeness, oneness, and well-being with the self and with the world in which the person now finds him/herself. These stages also describe the unfolding of the human task as the person seeks to find new meaning in a life that is coming to a close. As such, it is easy to see how each stage can appear, reappear, and appear in conjunction with other stages. What is presented here, therefore, is not so much the stages through which one may or may not pass during the process of dying but, more importantly to the intent of this book, how the person seeks to integrate the reality of death into his/her life, find meaning in that reality, and come to a sense of well-being in death.

Denial: "No, not me!" One psychological mechanism that appears in virtually all people who face the prospect of death is that of denial.[20] For Kübler-Ross, it is a stage that reappears throughout the dying process.[21] Denial is rooted in the need to put the current situation away for a moment to give the person a rest from the anxiety associated with the terminal illness. As Kübler-Ross states, no one can look at the sun all of the time; sometimes it is necessary to look away for a moment.[22]

Seen as such, denial can be a healthy way of dealing with an uncomfortable and painful situation that could extend for some time.[23] Denial acts as a buffer, allowing the person a moment of calm. Later, the person will be able to call on other, less radical defenses to deal with the crisis. In short, denial provides a method of gaining some control within the situation until such time as the person is able to deal effectively with the new circumstances of life.

> *Depending very much on how a patient is told, how much time he has to gradually acknowledge the inevitable happening, and how he has been prepared throughout life to cope with stressful situations, he will gradually drop his denial and use less radical defense mechanisms.[24]*

Denial can sometimes be selective. Kübler-Ross mentions instances in which a dying person may be very open with those family members or staff with whom he/she can discuss the illness, while at the same time avoiding the issue in the presence of those who cannot tolerate such a discussion or the thought of death. Other people make it clear that, although there is implicit acceptance of the diagnosis, denial is needed across the board to retain sanity. In these instances, too, denial is a tool used by the person to exercise some control within his/her environment.

Anger: "Why me?" When a person begins to deal directly with the reality of death, the emotional response that results is often anger at the realization that "I am dying." This anger can be difficult for family and staff because it is often expressed in an almost totally random fashion.

Although people who are dying become angry at many things, the anger is often directed at losing control within one's life as a result of the limitations imposed by the illness and the system of care. For example, some people will exhibit anger at those responsible for dietary decisions because of the loss of control over what will be eaten. Waiting for an answer to a call for assistance can also be a source of anger in a situation of dependence.

Anger needs to be expressed. Often, it is vented toward the family and care givers. Family visits may be judged as being too early or too late, with too many or not enough people. At other times, the anger will be directed at individuals for very subtle reasons. Sometimes, the more energetic and capable the visitor, the angrier is the patient. In the patient's words: "*You* can walk out of here; *you* can go home at five and see the kids; *you* go to work."[25] The anger, expressed at the individual, is really anger at what the person represents: life, functioning, and energy. Anger is expressed at all those things that the dying person is in the process of losing or has already lost.

Often, anger will be a direct response to care or to the lack of it. In a study to determine the time it took nurses to respond to a patient's call, it was discovered that patients who were terminally ill often had to wait twice as long as the others.[26] The frustration of being alive yet being treated as if already dead can be a great cause for anger as the person begins to feel abandoned. Some of this sense of abandonment springs from others who cannot or will not face death. Much of it results when those receiving the anger retreat; they take the anger personally instead of trying to discover its true meaning.

Bargaining: "Yes me, but . . ." Kübler-Ross' third stage of dying is bargaining. Bargaining consists quite simply of an attempt to arrange an agreement to postpone, if not cancel, the inevitable. Bargaining for more time can be as helpful as denial in gaining some distance from the prospect of death.

The purpose of bargaining is to attempt to gain some control through an effort to buy time. It generally consists of a commitment on the patient's part to perform some specific task if he/she will live until a certain date. This might be until a child is born, a wedding, or some other family event. It generally also includes a specific promise not to ask any more favors if this one last postponement is granted. It has been Kübler-Ross' experience that this promise is not kept.

Psychologically, this promised commitment may be associated with guilt and should not be ignored. For example, a commitment to dedicate one's remaining time in service to God in exchange for a longer life may spring from guilt over previous laxity toward religion. Guilt over events in one's past life must be resolved before an acceptance of the end of that life is possible.

Depression: "Oh! . . . Poor me." Depression often arises from the continued losses experienced throughout the illness. Physically, the person becomes weaker and more dependent on others and on machines. There are other losses as well, such as financial ones, the loss of a job or professional position, and the loss of relationships. Denial can serve to ward

71

off this depression for a time. Eventually, however, to one degree or another, the person must begin to deal with the losses brought on by the illness. Some form of depression will inevitably result as he/she begins to grieve these losses.

Kübler-Ross makes a distinction between two kinds of depression.[27] The first she refers to as "reactive depression." Reactive depression is brought on by the realization of loss in one's life. This form of depression is a natural response. In cases of reactive depression, the person is usually quite verbal and may find active intervention to facilitate a coming to terms with loss and a moving out of the depression.

The second type of depression to which Kübler-Ross refers is "preparatory depression." Preparatory depression occurs not over the past loss, but rather results from the anticipation of some impending loss. As such, it is .very similar to what Sourkes refers to as "anticipatory grief," which seeks to come to terms with a loss even before it is experienced.[28] Preparatory depression is a "tool to prepare for the impending loss of all the love objects in order to facilitate the state of acceptance."[29] In short, it is part of the person's efforts to cope with dying by preparing for the losses that will be entailed.

With preparatory depression, the person is usually quiet. There may be a tendency to tell the person to "cheer up." Kübler-Ross raises the question of why. The person's depression flows out of what is seen to be an unfortunate situation. Feelings of sadness are valid and understandable. This is a sad time for the person, and coping is better facilitated by allowing that person to express his/her sorrow rather than to deny it. There is no need for any psychiatric intervention. In fact, Kübler-Ross writes that many patients become angry when a psychiatric consultation is suggested because "they have dared to become depressed."[30] This depression is normal. It is necessary to remember that the person is occupied with things ahead, not behind. Preparatory depression "is necessary and beneficial if the patient is to die in a stage of acceptance and peace."[31]

Acceptance: "It's time." Acceptance is a very confused concept with respect to dying. Some equate it with a form of happiness; it is not. Others might think of acceptance as a kind of willingness to die; this is also not the case. There is no reason for the person to be either happy about the idea of dying or willing to leave behind family and friends. Acceptance has to do with integration, that is, coming to terms with the reality that the self is going to die. Although the person may not want to die, there is an element of peace in the realization that the person "can" die. It is not a moment of happiness because it is always sad that one has to leave in death. Although the person may not want to go, he/she nevertheless comes to a realization that, as one woman expressed it, "it is time to go."

Kübler-Ross is careful to draw a distinction between acceptance and resignation.[32] Resignation is a bitter giving up that flows out of an attitude of pessimism. This attitude, mentioned earlier, seeks to reconcile people with death by focusing on the futility of life. It is usually indignant, full of bitterness and anguish. There may be a sense of frustration and uselessness as the person seemingly throws up his/her arms in defeat to ask, "What's the use?"

Acceptance, on the other hand, involves a sense of "readiness to go."[33] It is in no way a contradiction to any positive attitude of the will that moves one to keep fighting for life. Acceptance of death is the most realistic goal that a person can work toward in view of the fact that everyone will die sooner or later. When a person has accepted the reality of his/her own finiteness, then that person has a much better chance of using one's internal energies to help the medical staff work to keep that person alive. Acceptance does not rule out life, but rather enhances the appreciation of life and the will to live fully.

Kübler-Ross sees two types of people who move to acceptance. The first is that person who will achieve it with little, if any, help from the outside. Perhaps the only need will be for silent understanding with no interference. This, she writes, is usually the older person who feels that life has been lived, the family has been raised, and he/she has completed life's tasks.[34] In fact, this can be anyone who is able to look back and put meaning and significance into one's life.

The others are those who need more active assistance as they struggle through the stages of denial, anger, bargaining, and depression. These stages, as already indicated, are part of a coping mechanism that allows the person to discover some meaning in what is happening. In this, the person moves toward an acceptance of one's own dying to a state of integration and well-being. Munley speaks of this time of transition as involving an inevitable tension between hanging on and letting go. It is, she writes, impossible to separate the dynamics of resignation and rejection from hope and acceptance in dying.[35] It is not surprising, then, to see the person move in and out of this moment of acceptance.

It has been observed that some people seem to regress emotionally after having begun to accept death. Much of this is not regression at all, but actually a misunderstanding by others of what is happening. Rather than regressing emotionally, the person is actually beginning to separate him/herself from the world. Kübler-Ross speaks of this period as a time when the patient begins to "wean off" life.[36] During this time, the person looks for fewer interpersonal relationships. As the end approaches, the person generally desires to maintain a relationship with only those who have been closest. Sourkes speaks of this as a process in which the one dying and the family flow between a sense of relatedness and a sense of letting go: "The patient, who is preparing for the loss of everything and everyone, gradually gives up the peripheral, while remaining ultimately attached to those closest."[37]

When there is an experience of some emotional regression, it most often has little to do with acceptance on the patient's part and much to do with the lack of acceptance by others. Sometimes the person is ready to let go whereas the family is not. In such a case, the family may need assistance in bringing the relationship to closure so that the person can be, as it were, "allowed" to die. Sourkes notes that a paradox often exists in these relationships. As the time of death draws near, the family, who is often better able to let go earlier in the illness, now feels less and less inclined to do so. At the same time, the person dying, who earlier sought to cling to life, is now moving toward a greater acceptance of death: "This is an anguished crossroads, for it indicates the recognition that the patient and family are moving in different directions."[38]

It is important to recognize that when a dying person has reached a genuine stage of acceptance yet does begin to show signs of emotional regression, this may be because those caring for the person do not allow him/her to let go. Unnecessary life-prolonging procedures that the person no longer appreciates may be introduced, or a family member may make the patient feel guilty for dying. It is in this last instance especially that an emotional regression is usually a sign of inappropriate care.

To illustrate this point is the case of a young woman who used to weep after visits by her husband. She confided that his visits troubled her because she was ready to die, but he insisted that she would get better and come home. Eventually, the husband was helped to join his wife in her acceptance. Her emotional state heightened, she became much more responsive to her care, and did return home again for one last visit. Other cases that illustrate how a lack of acceptance by others can influence the person dying often involve children. It has been noted that children suffering from a terminal disease sometimes seem not to die without some kind of permission, however subtle, from parents. Whether this is rooted in a child's need for permission or in a child's concern not to hurt or disappoint parents is not clear. What is clear is that for many, dying, which is already a difficult task, can be made more difficult by a lack of acceptance by others.

A CRITIQUE OF THE CONTEMPORARY VIEWS ON DEATH

This chapter began with an overview of some of the different ways in which humanity has tried to be reconciled with the reality of death. A close look revealed these to be ways of trying to get around death. Society's attempts to deal with death are often made by hiding it, putting it out of public view as much as possible. This hiding has led to many popular conceptions that, although they admit to the reality of death, deny the possibility of any kind of reconciliation with it. Death is seen as an evil to be avoided when possible. When this is not possible, the response of the survivors is simply to move on and hope for a better day tomorrow.

Having examined in some detail the subjective, personal experience of death, it is now possible to offer a critique of these conceptions. These are, in fact, fallacies. They deny that a person can be at one with him/herself as one who is dying and thus die well. They deny the possibility of what has been shown to be possible.

The first and third conceptions, that only suicidal and psychotic people want to die and that reconciliation with death is impossible, appear now to be merely excuses for the avoidance of death by the living. These conceptions offer reasons why the topic should never be mentioned and why people should not be told they are going to die. They allow family and care givers to distance themselves from an unpleasant reality by abandoning the dying person. This may be done emotionally and spiritually as well as physically. With this in mind, Kübler-Ross is convinced "that we do more harm by avoiding the issue than by using the time and timing to sit, listen, and share."[39]

The second conception, that the fear of death is one of the most basic fears, is also an excuse to avoid the reality of death. Although it is true that people do fear death, there are two dimensions to this fear: natural fears associated with death and learned fears.

When people are asked to describe their fears of death, they most often mention first the fears associated with pain and abandonment. Only later do people mention such fears as those involving the unknown or change. The ones that come to mind first are learned fears. People learn to fear death because their only experience of death, or others' experiences they have heard about, has been of death associated with pain and abandonment. Once these more repulsive fears are expressed, the healthier fears, those that actually seek to protect us from harm, come to the fore. These are fears that generally do not paralyze people. They raise a note of caution but do not generally dissuade a person from moving toward whatever may be feared. It might be said, then, that it is not so much death that is feared, but the manner in which people are allowed or made to die.

Some of the fears associated with death are most basic. Others, however, are learned. In the final analysis, it is the learned fears that move us away from accepting the reality of death. If they could be unlearned, the closer one comes to death, the lesser, not greater, the intensity of this fear would be.

The fourth conception, stating that a dying person never really wants to know, is based on the assumption that the person is unwilling to discuss death. It is wrong, however, to assume that someone who asks few questions has no interest. People know very well with whom they can and cannot talk. This was seen earlier in the discussion of selective denial. If the care giver does not allow for questions and discussion, then this will not happen. It is wrong to assume that this is the desire of the person when it may be the unconscious or even deliberate intent of the other.

In addition, when it comes to telling someone the truth about his/her situation, Kübler-Ross points out that the question is not so much "Should we tell?" as it is "How do we tell?"[40] People can tolerate even the most morbid of information when it is delivered in a loving manner and they know that the person giving them this information is not going to abandon them in their illness.

The fifth conception, which states that the person dying should be kept comfortable and allowed to withdraw and die in peace, is also based on incorrect assumptions. Withdrawal does not necessarily indicate peacefulness. Kübler-Ross was careful to point out the difference between reactive and preparatory depression. Both may appear to be the same, but they demand two different clinical responses to ensure that the person will continue to move toward acceptance. Even acceptance is deceptively similar in appearance to resignation, which contains more bitterness than peace.

This fallacy also assumes that suffering has to do primarily with the experience of pain. As was shown earlier and will be seen again in a discussion of pain in Chapter Four, this is not the case. Pain and suffering are not the same experience. Merely keeping the patient free from pain is not adequate care or assistance to one who is trying to get on with his/her dying. More needs to be done than keeping the person physically comfortable.

The sixth conception presupposes that survivors easily get over the death of a loved one; this is seldom the case. Bereavement can be a long and difficult process and can involve a suffering all its own. Some people express surprise at their feelings and at the pain and loneliness that comes from a death for which they thought they were prepared. Other people find themselves grieving for a loved one long after the death.

One example involves a student whose father died only days before the start of the academic year. Midway through the semester the student's grades began to drop, his ability to concentrate was hampered, and he found himself wanting to cry for no apparent reason. In counseling it became apparent that he was now, somewhat reluctantly, doing the grieving he did not have time to do when his father died. In another case involving a university student, a young woman's father died after a long illness. At the time, his death was experienced as relief by the surviving family members. At commencement, however, feelings of loss and grief emerged, much to the surprise and confusion of the young graduate. A final example concerns a middle-aged woman whose husband had died after a long illness. Since she had experienced many "little deaths" because of his illness, she and her family thought that she was prepared for the final one; she was not. Her grief at the time of his death surprised and frightened her and her family.

Grief must be expressed somehow and, when it is expressed, it should be validated and viewed as healthy, no matter how surprising or delayed after the death.

It is not unusual for survivors to experience serious physical and psychological symptoms during the first year or two after the death. The dying person's problems may come to an end, but the family's difficulties go on. Toynbee notes: "There are two parties to the suffering that death inflicts, the person dying and the survivors. In the apportionment of this suffering, the survivor takes the brunt."[41]

This sixth conception also speaks of an unnecessary suffering that should never be imposed on anyone. It may be asked, "Whose suffering is the focus of concern, the dying person's or the family's?" Suffering has been defined as the sense of being overwhelmed by some outside force over which one has no control. This sense is not dissipated by passive non-intervention. It can only be dealt with by an active acceptance of reality.

Reality should be faced as objectively as possible. Suffering will only be increased by the avoidance of the reality of death because the dying person and family will be unable to put meaning and order into it. Suffering does not lie in the dying but in the inability to make sense out of it. Well-being in death is not the equivalent of peace and tranquility, and well-being is not lacking where fear, pain, and disappointment exist. Dying well has to do with dying as a person and all that this entails.

The seventh conception, that the emotional and psychological sides of dying are overemphasized and that the physician is the central figure in the scenario of death, is also unfounded. Parkes insists that a knowledge of the psychological aspects of dying is as important to those who care for people approaching death as a knowledge of anatomy is to a surgeon.[42]

This is perhaps the most dangerous fallacy because it tends to reduce the person to a stereotype. Dying does not presuppose that personhood is already lost, such that the only need is to care for a body soon to be a corpse. Even in dying, the person must remain an active participant in his/her own care and living. The opportunities to control one's treatment, to maintain a sense of dignity, and to be as free as possible of pain should not be taken from a person simply because he/she is dying. The role of psychosocial or spiritual support may even take precedence over medical intervention.

RECONCILIATION WITH DEATH

For humanity in general, perhaps reconciliation with death is impossible. For a dying human being is particular, however, reconciliation is possible. The clinical observations of Kübler-Ross and others who have devoted their medical careers to understanding death, as well as my clinical experience, indicate that it is possible to be reconciled with one's own death. Reconciliation is possible and one's fears are allayed when the person is able to come to terms with and find meaning in what is happening:

> *For some people the greatest fear is that it is beyond their control and beyond their understanding, but the real fear which is repressed and unconscious is because of a view of death as a catastrophic destructive force and has ultimately to do with our own potential destructiveness. I believe if we could come to grips with our own destructiveness, we would then be able to overcome our own fear of death.*[43]

Reconciliation is just that: coming to terms with, rather than trying to get around, our own mortality. Reconciliation does not occur through attempts to put death off, to deny its existence, or even to say that it is of no consequence because it merely leads to some other reality that is better than this one.[44] Reconciliation results from the personal acceptance that each person will, one day, come to a point of death. Once the reality of death is accepted as part of who we are, then we can begin to face it.

Humanity confronts death by seeking to die well, by being at one with that moment of life. This is accomplished through coping—through the use of natural "tools" to come to terms with what is happening. Through this comes the knowledge that death is not the ultimate tragedy of life and that a person *can* die. Reconciliation has to do with coming to an acceptance of the reality, although not necessarily liking the reality, that human beings die.

Not a happy thought perhaps, but nevertheless a mature thought and one that invites life.

In looking at the ways people are reconciled with their own death, it is important not to equate "being ready to die" with "wanting to die." Being reconciled does not necessarily involve a desire to die, any more than acceptance must involve happiness. Being reconciled to death involves simply a knowledge and acceptance of reality because it has meaning.

This knowledge or acceptance is not so very different from the experience of moving out of the family home on reaching adulthood, moving away to or from school, or ending some childhood friendships. These, too, are called deaths or "little deaths," because it hurts to leave and, although one may not want to leave, he/she knows that the time has come. There are tears and heartache, but the move is made.

Biological death is not dissimilar. A person can come to a sense that, although staying is desired, it is time to move on. In this experience, a person is able to be reconciled with his/her own death, beyond what his/her philosophical or religious beliefs say about death in general. This would explain why people with no religious beliefs in an afterlife or no philosophy of life that seeks to explain death can die in peaceful acceptance, whereas others with thousands of years of religious tradition behind their beliefs remain afraid and unwilling to let go. Theories and beliefs can help humanity to be reconciled with mortality in general, but only the experience of being at one with oneself as a person who is dying and finding some personal meaning in that event can reconcile an individual to his/her own death. Regardless, and sometimes even in spite, of the presence or absence of faith or philosophy, people can be reconciled to the fact of their death.

In death, reconciliation involves being at one with the self as one who is dying. In this context, reconciliation has to do with dying well. This is not automatic and, as some of the clinical examples cited here indicate, can be disrupted. With support, however, it can happen. People go through natural stages or transitions that allow them to cope, to integrate, to find meaning, and to restore oneness—in short, to become well again even in their dying. Persons have the ability to be integrated with the self and the environment. This is no different in dying than it is in any other life experience. It may be more difficult, but it remains equally as possible, if it is allowed. To quote Shneidman:

You don't have to be anybody to die, and you shouldn't have to be highly placed in society to die well. It is obvious that one is more likely to die well if one has ego strength at the beginning of the trial and if one is lucky and has a good support system of loving people in one's life, and lastly, if that system *(including especially the way in which the art of medicine is practiced on you)* will let you. (emphasis added)[45]

The task is now to describe a system that allows this well-being.

NOTES

1. I contend that death is always subjective and personal. It is subjective in that it is one's own experience, and it is personal in that one always dies as a person in relation to the world, not as an individual without others. Dying is an experience of that whole person characterized in Chapter Two. It is important, therefore, to take note of the whole person in the dying process to understand its meaning for the person.
2. Elisabeth Kübler-Ross, *Death: The Final Stage of Growth,* Prentice-Hall, Englewood Cliffs, NJ, 1975.
3. Phillipe Ariès, "Five Variations on Four Themes," in *Death: Current Perspectives,* 3rd ed., ed. Edwin S. Shneidman, Mayfield Publishing, Palo Alto, CA, 1984, p. 62 (hence referred to as *Death: Current Perspectives).*
4. My own reflections are drawn from some of those presented by Arnold Toynbee, "Various Ways in Which Human Beings Have Sought to Reconcile Themselves to the Fact of Death," in *Death: Current Perspectives,* pp. 73-96.
5. Toynbee, p. 80.
6. William F. May, "Institutions as Symbols of Death," in *Death and Society: A Book of Readings and Sources,* eds. James P. Carse and Arlene B. Dallery, Harcourt Brace Jovanovich, New York, 1977, p. 411.
7. Geoffrey Gorer, "The Pornography of Death," in *Death: Current Perspectives,* p. 28.
8. Robert Nisbet, "Death," in *Death: Current Perspectives,* p. 120.
9. May, pp. 407-426.
10. See Avery D. Weisman, "Common Fallacies About Dying Patients," in *Death: Current Perspectives,* pp. 222-225.
11. For a discussion on the notion of the fear of death as being learned or innate, see Ernest Becker, "The Terror of Death," in *Death: Current Perspectives,* pp. 62-72.
12. Anne Munley, *The Hospice Alternative: A New Concept for Death and Dying,* Basic Books, New York, 1983, p. 145.
13. Barbara M. Sourkes, *The Deepening Shade: Psychological Aspects of Life-Threatening Illness,* University of Pittsburgh Press, Pittsburgh, 1982, p. 25.
14. Sourkes, p. 27.
15. C. Murray Parkes, "Psychological Aspects," in *The Management of Terminal Disease,* ed. Cicely M. Saunders, Edward Arnold Publishers Ltd., London, 1978, p. 47.

16. Elisabeth Kübler-Ross, *On Death and Dying*, Macmillan, New York, 1969; "What is it like to be dying?" in *The American Journal of Nursing* 71, 1971, pp. 54-61; *Questions and Answers on Death and Dying*, Macmillan, New York, 1974; *Living with Death and Dying*, Macmillan, New York, 1981; *Death: The Final Stage of Growth*.

17. See, for example, Robert J. Kastenbaum, *Death, Society, and Human Experience*, 3rd ed., The C.V. Mosby Co., St. Louis, 1985, pp. 209-213; John B. Williamson, *Aging and Society*, Holt, Rinehart & Winston, New York, 1980, pp. 333-335; Loma Feigenberg, *Terminal Care: Friendship Contracts with Dying Cancer Patients*, trans. Patrick Hort, Brunner/Mazel, New York, 1980; and Richard Schulz and David Aderman, "Clinical Research and the Stages of Dying," *Omega 5*, 1974, pp. 137-143.

18. Edwin S. Shneidman, "Some Aspects of Psychotherapy in Dying Persons," in *Death: Current Perspectives*, especially p. 275.

19. Kübler-Ross, *Questions and Answers on Death and Dying*, p. 25.

20. Avery D. Weisman, *On Dying and Denying: A Psychiatric Study of Terminality*, Behavioral Publications, New York, 1972.

21. Kübler-Ross, *On Death and Dying*, p. 38.

22. Kübler-Ross, *On Death and Dying*, p. 39.

23. See also Richard S. Lazarus, "Positive Denial: The Case for Not Facing Reality," *Psychology Today* 13, 1979, pp. 44-60.

24. Kübler-Ross, *On Death and Dying*, p. 42.

25. Kübler-Ross, "What is it like to be dying?" pp. 57-58.

26. Kübler-Ross, p. 57.

27. Kübler-Ross, pp. 86-111.

28. Sourkes, p. 67; see also C. Knight Aldrich, "Some Dynamics of Anticipatory Grief," in *Anticipatory Grief*, eds. Bernard Schoenberg *et al.* Columbia University Press, New York, 1974, p. 4.

29. Kübler-Ross, *On Death and Dying*, p. 87.

30. Kübler-Ross, "What is it like to be dying?" p. 58.

31. Kübler-Ross, *On Death and Dying*, p. 87.

32. Kübler-Ross, *Questions and Answers on Death and Dying*, p. 25.

33. Kübler-Ross, "What is it like to be dying?" p. 58.

34. Kübler-Ross, *On Death and Dying*, p. 49.

35. Munley, pp. 155-156.

36. Kübler-Ross, *Questions and Answers on Death and Dying*, p. 13.

37. Sourkes, p. 75.

38. Sourkes, p. 69.

39. Kübler-Ross, *On Death and Dying*, p. 142.

40. Kübler-Ross, *On Death and Dying*, p. 142.

41. Arnold Toynbee, "The Relation Between Life and Death, Living and Dying," in *Death: Current Perspectives*, p. 14.

42. Parkes, p. 44.

43. Kübler-Ross, *Questions and Answers on Death and Dying*, p. 156.

44. I do not mean here to deny the reality of a rebirth, a life after death, a resurrection of the dead, the existence of a heaven and hell, or any other belief

in a kind of continued existence after physical death. Rather, I am suggesting that any such belief is not a sine qua non for the acceptance on one's own death. This acceptance does not depend on, may not be rooted in, or may not even be made easier by a belief in some afterlife.
45. Schneidman, p. 283.

4 / *Palliative Care*

The preceding discussion of the person, the meaning of well-being and suffering, and the goals of medicine has been for the purpose of understanding more fully the notion of palliative care for the terminally ill. The purpose of this chapter is to define and illustrate that modality within the full context of medical care.

This chapter will begin with a definition of palliative care and a discussion of its place within medicine. To illustrate the distinctiveness of palliative care, a description of the care setting will be included. The model used here is the Palliative Care Unit at Western Massachusetts Hospital in Westfield, MA. Through this description, the tone and style of care become more apparent.

The second section will focus on symptom control. Although palliative care is not synonymous with symptom control or with terminal care per se,[1] this is the medical reality of principal concern here. Before doing this, it will first be necessary to define what it means to say that someone is terminally ill.

The focus of the third section will be therapy. With respect to cancer, the three principal modes of therapy—surgery, radiation therapy, and chemotherapy—will be discussed. The comparison of these therapies in both aggressive and palliative settings will help to illustrate their distinctiveness in practice and will clarify the appropriateness and inappropriateness of each modality in different care settings. The treatment of acquired immune deficiency syndrome (AIDS) must be, of necessity, somewhat different.

In the treatment of AIDS, there is no curative therapy and, as will be seen, aggressive therapy is generally directed not so much toward the AIDS virus itself as it is toward the opportunistic infections that result as a consequence of the person's suppressed immune system. Although there may be hope in the treatment of cancer to allow for a slowing or even remission of the disease process, therapy associated with AIDS, at present, is much more of a defensive response to complications as they arise. For this reason, the discussion of AIDS will address not only surgery, radiation, and chemotherapy, but also the treatment of opportunistic infections. Although the section on cancer will give insight into the distinctiveness of palliative care, the discussion of AIDS therapy will serve principally to illustrate the rationale for moving away from aggressive therapy and toward palliative care.

Two areas of symptom control will require particular attention, one because of its centrality to the principle of palliation and the other because of its controversial nature. These are the issues of pain control and the maintaining of adequate nutritional and hydrational levels.

The control of physical pain is central. Unless the person is free from pain, or at least from the anxiety so often associated with it, other attempts to relieve the person's suffering will be of little benefit. With regard to the question of "feeding" a patient, there is a great deal of discussion and little agreement within the medical profession, ethical writings, and public policy in the United States. The question is whether maintaining normal levels of nutrition or hydration is a basic human right that can never be refused or denied, or a therapeutic measure that, like other therapies, can be withheld or withdrawn when it offers no reasonable hope of benefit. Because of the complexities involved in both pain control and nutritional support, each of these issues will be treated in separate sections and at greater length than the other palliative modalities.

PALLIATIVE CARE DEFINED

The word *palliative* is derived from the Latin *palliare,* meaning "to cloak." Mount speaks of palliation as meaning "to improve the quality of."[2] Palliative care, therefore, has to do with the covering of symptoms with the intent of relieving distress in order that a person may be as free as possible to enjoy life within the limits of some disease, thereby improving the quality of that life.

In cases of illness when the possibility of a cure exists, attempts are made to relieve distressing symptoms. Palliation in this instance is an aspect of acute care.[3] As members of the medical profession seek to cure an individual, they do so partly by relieving distressing symptoms. Although it is certainly possible that the person could suffer prolonged health impairment or even death if left untreated, in this case the reasonable hope exists that aggressive treatment will lead to a cure. Palliation of symptoms is in service to that goal of cure.

Cases of chronic illness also involve palliation, which may extend for long periods.[4] The goal of chronic medical treatment is to prolong a person's life while, at the same time, maintaining an acceptable quality of life within the limits of the circumstances. In these instances, the person is not faced with a condition that will result in death, at least not in the predictable future or without the development of some further complications. Palliation of symptoms serves the goal of prolonging life with as much personal integrity as possible.

There are many people, however, for whom acute care seems inappropriate because a cure is not possible. There are also people for whom chronic care seems inappropriate; their condition is such that, although life can be prolonged, it can only be done at the expense of unacceptable losses with respect to the quality of one's life. Finally, there are people who are actively dying; their condition is at times referred to as "hopeless," and it is often believed that nothing more can be done for them. These people are in need of an approach to healthcare that has a different goal. They seek neither a cure nor a prolonging of life. Instead, they seek the relief of distress with the purpose of maintaining as high a quality of life as possible in the time remaining. This is palliative care. The goal is neither "return" nor "more time." The goal is simply "well-being today."

A description of palliative care as one of three modalities of healthcare—acute care, chronic care, and palliative care—will illustrate this point more clearly.

Acute Care

Acute care is that mode of care necessitated by the presence of an illness or injury that affects a person over a period of less than six to eight months, with full recovery expected with little or no residual impairment.[5] For example, a young man may suffer an acute myocardial infarction. This man will be placed in the acute care setting of the cardio-care unit of a local hospital. With good care, and if the damage to the heart is minimal or nonexistent, he can hope to return to his previous state of health, to his family, to work, and, in the context of the human task model, to a new beginning of life.

Chronic Care

There are times when cure is not a realistic goal of medicine. In these instances, the person finds him/herself in a chronic care situation typified by the presence of some disease or injury that persists longer than six to eight months, with any recovery being partial and usually associated with some degree of impairment or disability.[6] The goal of medicine in this instance is one of prolonging life through the modification of one's body and/or life style. An example might be a diabetic person who requires the amputation of a limb because of poor circulation. Although the person's life may be threatened by the gangrenous situation in the limb brought on by the poor circulation resulting from the diabetes, the diabetes itself does not directly threaten the life of the person. The person's medical crisis arises from a complication derived from, but not necessarily inherent to, the primary disease. The disease cannot be cured, but the crisis can be relieved through the amputation. The person will require surgery and psychological and physical therapy but can live many more years with an acceptable quality of life as a result of the modification. Again, within the context of the human task, the person can move on to further growth and development.

Palliative Care

In each of these medical situations, there is a concern for the future. When the goal of cure is no longer realistic, or when the balance between length of life and acceptable quality of life is lost, there is a shift away from the future and toward the present. This is the focus of palliative care. The goal of medicine here shifts from *more life* to *living well*. The patient is dying, but the focus is not so much on the reality of death as it is on the act of dying. That is, the focus is on the quality of life remaining and the well-being of the person who is engaged in the human task of bringing closure to life.

If death is viewed as some force that overtakes people from the outside, then such care makes no sense. Death, as an evil force, should always be kept at bay. As stated earlier, however, this is not a realistic understanding of death. Death is not so much something that happens *to* people as it is something people *do*. Death is an event in life that is lived out. Dying is a living experience. Palliative care takes as its foundation the reality that the dying process is irreversible and that death is imminent. The reality of the situation dictates that to speak of cure is deceptive, and to modify will merely prolong without improvement and may contribute to suffering. Palliative care bases itself on the premise that life is not so much to be prolonged as it is to be lived, and that bringing life to closure is part of living. There is a shift toward living as fully as possible the time left today without seeking to make more tomorrows. The goal is to heighten quality and to achieve well-being even at the risk of shortening quantity.

A Philosophy of Palliative Care

It is imperative that the distinction between acute, chronic, and palliative care, as well as the movement from one to another, be recognized. This is particularly true in view of the fact that approximately two thirds of all people who die will move into a situation in which the goal should be to improve the quality of time left without necessarily seeking to prolong it.[7] Saunders shows this movement in her "cure" and "care" system diagram illustrated in Fig. 4.1.[8]

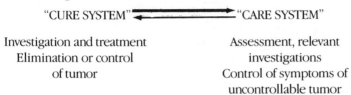

"CURE SYSTEM" ⟷ "CARE SYSTEM"

| Investigation and treatment Elimination or control of tumor | Assessment, relevant investigations Control of symptoms of uncontrollable tumor |

Fig. 4.1 Saunders' Cure System–Care System

Where there are different goals, there will be a different application of medical therapies. Likewise, there may be a different ethical reasoning for the determination of the appropriateness of medical intervention. As aggressive treatment becomes increasingly irrelevant, a movement is made toward palliative therapy. However, no one should ever be locked irreversibly into what is or may become an inappropriate care setting. Although these are distinct, they are not mutually exclusive. This can be seen in the "two-way" dimension of Saunders' diagram. Just as palliation has a place in acute and chronic care, the aggressive principles of these latter two may be sometimes applicable to the person with a terminal disease. This may be especially true of the person with AIDS who is just beginning to develop, or has shown a good potential to recover from, opportunistic infections. Further, as methods of treatment become more effective, the distinction becomes less clear. Care settings, therefore, should not be applied too rigidly. What is important to establish is that the person is in the appropriate care setting, receiving appropriate care, at each stage of the illness or recovery. This might be determined in part by posing the question, "Where is this person in the pursuit of his/her own human task?"

One could get the impression that acute and chronic care are "active" medical interventions whereas palliative care is "passive." Part of this conception is rooted in the common notion that there is nothing that can be done for one who is dying and that the situation is hopeless. In fact, this is not the case. Even in situations of death, it is seldom, if ever, true that nothing helpful can be done. It will only seem that nothing more can be done if care is cure oriented or if time is seen as a necessary complement to life. People who are dying are generally too realistic to expect that the medical staff can take away what is happening. What they do expect is concern and care for their distress and symptoms as they seek to be at one with their dying. As has already been illustrated, there are many such symptoms and elements of distress. Palliative care is more than handholding. It involves the active and expert involvement of an interdisciplinary team made up of specialists in chemotherapy, radiation, surgery, anesthesiology, physical therapy, social and spiritual services, and psychosocial and nutritional support who work together to help bring the dying person to a sense of well-being.[9]

Palliative care also addresses a prevailing misunderstanding of terminal care. Dunphy makes reference to this misunderstanding by noting what he refers to as "misguided cries" for euthanasia on the one hand and threatened lawsuits for passive murder or neglect on the other.[10] Palliative care is rooted in the understanding that well-being can be achieved even for the person who is dying. Well-being is not served if the person's ability to be at one with him/herself as one who is dying is taken away. The person must exercise some control within his/her life situation if he/she is to achieve well-being. Palliative care seeks to assist in the attainment of well-being by giving the person this control. It would be counterproductive and therefore wrong to take this control away from the person, whether by medical denial of the situation and the introduction of curative care when cure is not possible or by taking over the dying process through euthanasia. At the same time, palliative care is the antithesis, not the legitimation, of neglect. The control of symptoms, particularly of pain, demands an expertise and an attention to detail that can and sometimes does supersede that found in acute or chronic care settings.[11]

It has been suggested that palliative care is appropriate for those who experience a shift away from the future and toward the present—appropriate for those whose healthcare goal has become the quality and not the length of life. It may be tempting to see the criteria for this appropriateness as being determined by time, that is, appropriate for the person with a limited number of days or weeks to live. This is not necessarily the case. In fact, how much time is left should not be the determining factor primarily because this is difficult to predict. Advanced metastatic disease is not a reliable index of terminal illness.[12] It is not always possible to predict its precise course or outcome. This is particularly true of progressive diseases such as cancer and AIDS. In addition to the clinical variables, there are often personal variables as well. Clinical evidence has shown that some people will seemingly refuse to die until their affairs are in order, regardless of the prognosis.

In spite of this, it is common to hear of medical personnel who give a fixed number of months or a year for the person to live. This is the person for whom it is often assumed that palliative care is now appropriate. Dunphy writes that to make a statement that an individual will only live for a given time is "unforgiveable because there are no valid grounds for so rigid a prognosis. . . . One can never tell."[13] Kübler-Ross makes this same point:

I think it is the worst possible management of any patient, no matter how strong, to give him a concrete number of months or years. Since such information is wrong in any case, and exceptions in both directions are the rule, I see no reason why we even consider such information.[14]

To speak with such certainty, as if to put the person on some sort of schedule, reinforces the notion that death is something outside the person, lurking around the corner as it were, waiting for the right moment to pounce on its victim. Predictions can forget that death does not come for people, but that people die. In doing so, it can take away hope in the face of dying, a hope that exists in spite of the gravity of the situation. There is no false optimism, no promise of a cure stated explicitly by the physician or implicitly through therapy in palliative care. There is only the truth of the situation. When the truth is unencumbered by the frustration of the inability to make accurate predictions and the futile attempts to apply statistics to the individual person, there is hope for life even when one knows that he/she is dying. Truth gives hope that the person will not be abandoned and will be able to live out and find meaning in one's death.

Hope remains alive, but not in a hope for a cure or more time. Often it is presumed that people who are dying hope for an extended life. In reality, they are usually too ill or tired to hope for that. Hope does not always have an object. It may be a kind optimism that is part of the human spirit. This optimism can be suppressed by fear, pain, and suffering. If these can be controlled, then hope can endure. What the person hopes for is to pursue the human task of closure. Palliative care seeks to control pain and suffering to allow that optimism to come through in the person's life. In short, the anxiety of dying is eased so that the person can live in hope, a true hope of living in a meaningful way for whatever time is left.

Truth and hope are not mutually exclusive. Hope depends on truth and is lost, not gained, by deceptive attempts to deny the truth or to express it in a precise prognosis that will probably prove to be wrong. Palliative care seeks to maintain hope on the part of the one who is dying by accepting the reality of the situation and assisting the person in his/her attempt to be at one with it and to live it out with a sense of well-being. That does not involve a schedule one should follow.

The appropriateness of palliative care, therefore, is not determined by how much time may or may not be left. Rather, it is determined by the limitations of the capabilities of available modalities of therapy. The inability to be cured is not the failure of the person. It results from the limitedness that is part of human nature and inherent in medical therapies. In acute or chronic care, the person may die without treatment. Palliative care becomes appropriate when curative therapies are no longer viable, since the person is going to die even with treatment. Palliative care is appropriate when cure orientation is no longer realistic and when the paramount issue is the quality that can be put into living.

There are, then, three care settings in which a person may find him/herself in a health crisis. Each care setting has its own goals and, although each may share modalities of therapy, the implementation and expectation of those modalities will differ. Each has its own ethical underpinnings that speak of the appropriateness of care. In the acute care setting, the goal of medicine and the definition of well-being will involve a return to a previous state. In the chronic care setting, the goal will be the prolonging of life through modification of one's life situation, whether physical, psychological, spiritual, or psychosocial. Well-being will be found in the ability of the person to integrate him/herself with this new situation. In the palliative care setting, curative therapy is viewed as no longer appropriate because cure is not possible; prolonging of life will be viewed as no longer appropriate because longer life can only be achieved at the unacceptable sacrifice of the possible quality of the time that is left. Palliative care, therefore, is the expert and attentive interdisciplinary care of the person, through symptom control as well as emotional, spiritual, and psychosocial support, as that person lives out a limited time of life in the effort to achieve or maintain a state of well-being, rooted in the hope of living in a meaningful way with his/her dying.

The Unit of Palliative Care

Healthcare facilities such as acute and chronic care hospitals and clinics are established for curing a person of some affliction or for providing whatever supports are necessary to prolong life within a particular health need setting. To accomplish this, personnel, administration, and procedures are established that set the tone for care. Machines and facilities are available in sufficient quantities to provide required services.

Palliative care has as its goal the heightening of the quality of life of the dying person, assisting that person in attaining well-being in his/her present life situation. The palliative care unit is not a place of death, although people do die there. It is first and foremost a place of life and living, a place where people bring closure to their physical existence. It is a place of transition. Because the goals are different, so, too, is the facility.

Acute and chronic healthcare facilities, to be effective, need to focus on disease, trauma, and therapy to give the most effective care to the person. This same attention is needed in palliative care, yet the focus shifts more toward the person afflicted with the disease, injured in the trauma, or participating in the therapy. The person is dying, and the person needs care and attention. It is not so much that these are lacking in acute and chronic care facilities, but that the emphasis is different. In acute care, the person needs a sanitary setting. When a person is dying, he/she may have needs that might be thought of as being unsanitary, such as a pet dog lying on the end of the bed as it would at home. When someone is receiving care meant to get that person home as soon as possible, it is not important what the room looks like. When people are going to die and care at home is not possible, it is important that home come to them. This can be done by moving photos, a favorite chair, pillow, or other object into the unit. When critically ill, people need a physician's attention and rest; when dying, people sometimes need their spouse or lover in the bed with them or perhaps on a cot in the same room.

This subtle shift in emphasis calls for a rather major shift in the environment, new procedures, and different machines. The setting must be one that allows people to feel at home in their transition. The palliative care unit seeks to provide this setting. It is difficult to merely designate two or three beds in an acute care hospital for this purpose. It is difficult for the same nursing staff, for example, to engage in different modalities of care on the same corridor. The philosophy of care is different and can introduce tensions. Ideally, a palliative care unit should be established in a setting where procedural and philosophical tensions will not arise. This may be accomplished with a separate unit in a hospital or a free-standing independent facility.

The palliative care setting that I will use as an example in this work is the Palliative Care Unit (PCU) at Western Massachusetts Hospital, Westfield, MA. This unit is similar to other palliative care units and hospices throughout the United States and Canada. The PCU is a self-contained unit within a chronic care facility operated by the Department of Public Health of the Commonwealth of Massachusetts.

Western Massachusetts Hospital opened in 1910 as a hospital for the treatment of tuberculosis patients. In the 1950s, it became a research center for cancer treatment and was the site of many experimental procedures in radiation, surgery, and chemotherapy. Today, in addition to the PCU, Western Massachusetts Hospital has a 19-bed chronic care unit for the elderly, two

17-bed coma care units, and a pediatric unit for children with multiple handicaps and postdrowning trauma.

The PCU is a 17-bed unit devoted to the care of terminally ill persons and their families. This is perhaps one of the most important aspects of a palliative care facility: the unit of care is not simply the patient, but the patient/family. Often the family has information that is helpful to the staff in caring for the patient, and their active participation in care is necessary. They will know, better than the staff, the patient's hopes and how the disease has changed them and their outlook. All this information is needed to help the patient come to terms with his/her own dying.

Further, anything that affects the patient will affect the family, and vice versa. As the patient approaches death, the family will somehow be influenced, and this will be communicated to the patient in some manner. The family's fears, grief, and anxiety will be communicated to the patient, who may begin to feel a sense of failure at abandoning the family. Some families need to give the person who is dying a kind of permission, letting him/her know that they will be all right. Reconciliation between family members and the patient may be needed to assist the patient to die in peace and to prevent guilt on the part of some family members after death.

Illness and death always take place within the context of relationships, and all these must be cared for. Craven and Wald use the analogy of a mobile to explain the shifts within these relationships:

> *A family group can be compared to a mobile made up of infinite numbers and kinds of members suspended from a single strand. Each member can move and change independently to some degree, but every shift cannot help but precipitate movement of every other member and the whole.*[15]

Each relational shift must be noted in the care of the person who is dying. Ignore the needs of the family members, and management of the patient's needs will be compromised.

The PCU itself is T shaped. Along the vertical corridor is a meditation room, simply furnished with an altar/table and a bench along the back wall. This carpeted room with stained-glass windows remains primarily an open space to allow easy access for wheelchairs and beds. The room offers a setting for religious services, a quiet space to pray or simply "to be," as people struggle to find meaning in and be at one with their life. Books containing the Scriptures, inspirational writings, and thoughts on death and grieving can also be found here.

Across the hall is located the pastoral care office. Although not everyone believes in a God, an individual's transcendent nature is part of his/her being. Care for the person must include care for this as well. The spiritual or transcendent needs of the dying and their families often become critical during a terminal illness. Reconciliation with God, faith community, and family can often times be facilitated through pastoral care, which is often different from that found in acute care settings.

It is the practice in the Roman Catholic Church of the United States, for example, to anoint patients with the Oils of the Sick upon admission to a hospital or nursing home. This "sacrament of initiation" into a healthcare facility is inappropriate, particularly in a setting for the terminally ill. By its very nature, the sacrament celebrates reconciliation, something that is not automatically achieved simply through an anointing. Pastoral care in the PCU is personal as well as sacramental. The sacraments are never dispensed in a routine fashion. Care is always taken that they be the celebration of a spiritual reality. People are anointed only when they want to be. That may be on arrival, in the last moments of life, or not at all.

How even the sacraments or rituals of a faith community are a part of, and perhaps find their full meaning in, the pursuit of well-being in dying can be illustrated in two antithetical examples. In the first, I was asked to go to the PCU to offer assistance to a man who was dying with great difficulty and to his family. On arrival, I was informed that he was unresponsive. In his room, I stood on one side of his bed with his family on the other. He was lying on his side, facing his family. Knowing that he had been away from the Church for some time, I asked him if he wanted to be anointed. He responded by rolling over to me and grasping my hands. I suggested that we all join hands and pray the Lord's Prayer, after which I anointed him. He died before I had finished.

In the second case, involving another minister, a woman had told the pastoral care coordinator on admission that she did not want to be visited by anyone from her church. By chance, a local clergyman did stop in her room one day while visiting another patient. He entered the room, greeted the woman, said a prayer over her, and departed. After this visit, the woman began to experience nightmares and told the pastoral care coordinator that she believed she was going to hell. From that time on, her pain was never again adequately controlled. Clearly, all aspects of care must be sensitive to the needs of the one who is dying and do not have an absolute value or meaning simply in themselves.

People do not come to the PCU merely to die; they come to live. This is done, in part, through celebrations of life, such as birthday and holiday parties. These events always include the patients and their families. Other, more personal celebrations include anniversaries or weddings of family members. Games are coordinated to facilitate socialization among the patients and among their families. In short, an environment is created where the people become friends with and begin to care about each other.

Some patients may come together to play cards on a regular basis, visit each other in their rooms, and grieve for one another at the time of death. Families, too, become part of one another's lives, sharing each other's concerns. It often happens that some members of a family will continue to visit patients they have come to know in the PCU even after their own loved one has died.

This same corridor has two bedrooms, fully equipped with comfortable furniture, for use by the family. As the time of death approaches, some family members wish to remain. There are no posted visiting hours at the PCU, allowing family and friends of any age to come and go according to their needs and the needs of the patient.[16] When the hour or the situation makes staying overnight important, these rooms are available. Family members who wish to be closer to their loved one are given cots so that they can sleep in the patient's room. These bedrooms also make it possible for couples to share a little more privacy with each other in cases where the patient is too ill to leave the unit.

All the facilities of the PCU are shared equally with the family, and this is perhaps seen best in the kitchenette. Here is found a refrigerator, always stocked with cold drinks. Also available are coffee and tea, along with cookies and other snacks. The refrigerator is available to everyone to keep favorite, ethnic, or homemade foods. A microwave oven is available to heat up whatever the family has brought to the patient whenever he/she desires to eat. Always a place of activity, the kitchen table becomes an important place for all to share a cup of coffee and a friendly, supportive conversation among family, friends, and staff. As in most homes, it is here that most family support takes place.

Most of the meals in the PCU come from the main kitchen. Whereas any institutional kitchen must run on a schedule, efforts are made to have a meal ready when it is wanted. The microwave oven in the kitchenette is used frequently to reheat a meal after it is prepared. Each patient is given a wide range of choices on the menu, although most wish merely soup and a sandwich because of the effects of disease and therapy on a person's appetite. A dietician is on staff at the hospital to assist in the patient's care. The dietician meets with the patient to determine likes and dislikes, foods that are well tolerated, and so forth. In this way, a diet is planned that invites the person to eat, a diet in service to the person's psychological as well as nutritional needs. One woman, for example, ate scallops for lunch every day, seven days a week; she said she liked them and would miss them.

For special occasions, the kitchen prepares special meals: turkey on Thanksgiving or ham at Easter. Every effort is made to keep the menu as flexible and as important as it would be if the person were at home. Eating is a social event, and the normal hospital practice of eating alone or having others watch while the patient eats detracts from this. At the PCU, family members are always welcome to join the patient at any meal.

The nurses' station is found at the end of this corridor. Literally, it is the center of care, with the patients' rooms being found in either direction along the horizontal corridor of the T shape. Unlike most stations in typical acute care facilities, this one is open and spacious. Even patients in wheelchairs can enter. The large round table makes staff meetings easy and friendly. Between shifts, the staff meets here to review each patient. The patient's physical condition and medication as well as his/her psychosocial condition are noted to allow the oncoming shift to most effectively tend to his/her current needs. The nurses often do not wear standard uniforms, choosing instead to wear casual clothes that lend an air of friendliness.

Each patient's room is as different as the person in it. Each single room is equipped with a hospital bed, often with a water mattress to avoid pressure sores, and a dresser. After that, it is up to the patient. Some bring in a television or a radio, others a pet hamster, or an assortment of flowering or vegetable plants they wish to care for. Pictures and greeting cards hang on the walls, and afghans lie across beds and chairs, giving each room its own color, its own life.

Whereas a patient can request a phone in an acute care facility, these rooms do not have their own phone. Instead, the unit has a portable phone, and each room is equipped with a telephone jack. This practice helps provide greater privacy for the patient. Phone calls can often be untimely for someone who is ill, especially for a person who naps at different times throughout the day. All calls come in to the desk at the nurses' station and, if the person is awake and wants the call, the phone is brought to the room.

At the far end of the corridor is the day room. A place for gatherings and entertainment, this spacious and sunny room has an abundance of plants, a television, stereo, an aquarium, a library of paperbacks, and a treasury of games. Patients come here to read, to knit, to enjoy each other's or families' company, or simply to get out of their rooms for a while and enjoy the view. Western Massachusetts Hospital sits on 190 acres of open and wooded land. There are picnic tables and grills, flowering trees, a duck pond, and wooded paths where patients and families are free to enjoy the outdoors.

A whole range of services are offered at the PCU. For example, there are beauticians available for those patients who desire this service. Social workers, a clinical psychologist, and volunteer care givers (VCGs) assist patients and their families in various ways. An oncologist is available in the unit three days a week and is on call 24 hours a day. A urologist, whose services are needed frequently for assistance with catheters or in cases of bladder tumors, is also on call.

Western Massachusetts Hospital also makes available physical, occupational, speech and communication disorder, and respiratory therapy,[17] as well as an adult day care facility. There are also dental, optical, laboratory, and radiology facilities. Minor surgery with a local anesthetic, such as the drainage of an abscess, can be performed at the hospital. Outpatient surgery, radiation, and chemotherapy are available through nearby facilities when appropriate.

Death within the PCU is not the hidden event it sometimes is within society. Family members are left alone or joined by someone from the staff at the patient's bedside, as they wish. Although the door to the patient's room is usually closed, this is for privacy and not for the purpose of keeping death from anyone. Other patients often know when someone is dying and discuss it with the staff. After someone has died, other patients, particularly those who were friendly with the deceased, are informed. Family members may stay as long as they wish with the body. No effort is made to dress up the body of the deceased for viewing by the family. The care that the person has received makes such a dressing unnecessary.

Although it is seldom requested, it is possible for family members to have a special viewing of the body at the PCU. This is done in the meditation room. Most often, however, the body is transferred to a funeral home where final arrangements are made for services and a burial. Someone from the staff of the PCU, usually someone who has become close to the patient and/or the family during his/her stay at the PCU, visits the funeral home during the visiting hours or attends the service if there is one. The meditation room has been used on occasion for services when the patient has no family and has made such a request. For those with no home, the PCU becomes home. For these people, it is appropriate that some committal service be in the place where they found acceptance.

The patient/family is the unit of care. This means that, when death occurs, part of the unit of care remains. To be of assistance to the bereaved, the PCU offers support coordinated by a bereavement team made up of people from social service, psychology, and pastoral care. Part of this care is in the form of support groups for the bereaved and those preparing for the death of a loved one. These groups provide a place where people can express grief, listen, share, and learn from each other's experiences. They offer the opportunity to have feelings of loss, anger, or confusion validated. As people learn more about the events of dying and grief, they are better able to understand what is happening in their lives.

Within two weeks of the death, and again at three months, six months, and a year later, a card is sent to the family as a reminder of continued care and concern for them. A grief assessment is made in most cases in an effort to predict who will be in need and how they can best be helped in their grief. For the staff, too, assistance is given in the grieving process. Memorial services are held in the meditation room. These services allow staff members the opportunity to bring closure to the relationships they have shared with those for whom they have cared.

What one sees in this or any PCU is a specialized, interdisciplinary team coming together in a homelike setting. The hospitality of the unit allows patients to settle in quickly, usually within 24 to 48 hours. The unit allows the patients to take charge of their affairs as they prepare for death and gives families the support they will need to prepare for and live after death occurs. Its purpose is not that of acute or chronic care, and the setting reflects that difference. The PCU is a place of life and quality living, a place that, by its simple presence, offers hope to those who do not have long to live.

SYMPTOM CONTROL IN TERMINAL ILLNESS

Before symptom control or palliative care for the terminally ill person can be fully appreciated, it is first necessary to have an adequate understanding of a terminal disease. Although it is true that an important moment is reached when it is determined that a patient will no longer derive positive benefit from continued conventional treatment,[18] it is inaccurate to say that, at this point, the person is in a terminal state. Likewise, it is incorrect to say that having a disease, which by its very nature is terminal, makes the person with such a disease terminally ill. There are other factors involved that must be taken into account in an understanding of what it means to be terminally ill.

Terminal Illness

Medically, a diagnosis of a terminal illness is made after a careful assessment of the nature of the individual patient's symptoms, the evidence of an advanced and progressive disease, the inability to treat the disease by conventional means or the failure of these in a specific situation, and the psychological attitude of the patient. This is done only with a degree of difficulty. For example, a patient may complain of severe and incapacitating pain, yet have no rapidly progressive disease or show any evidence of clinical deterioration. At the same time, a patient may have an advanced, progressive disease and yet remain reasonably well, being able to work and function in a more or less normal fashion. Part of the difficulty lies in the fact that an advanced metastatic disease such as cancer or AIDS is not, in itself, a reliable index of terminal illness. A patient may remain stable for long periods even in the advanced stages of a terminal disease.

The failure of conventional treatment does not automatically mean that the person is now to be considered terminally ill. In many instances, when conventional treatment offers no chance of a cure, it can be very effective in extending the person's life. This will be seen in more detail in a later section. The mere failure of treatment to cure, therefore, does not constitute the condition of terminal illness.

At the same time, not everyone who contracts a disease that by its nature is terminal can be said to be terminally ill. The case of Kaposi's sarcoma, a tumor of the soft tissues, illustrates this point.

The North American strain of Kaposi's sarcoma, often referred to today as classic Kaposi's sarcoma (CKS), affects men over age 65 and runs a 20-year course. Although the disease is terminal, the person is not said to be terminally ill because he is more likely to die of old age or some other complication before age 85. Since 1985, however, Kaposi's sarcoma has been diagnosed in young men whose immune system has become depressed. In this context, it is referred to as epidemic Kaposi's sarcoma (EKS) and is one of the opportunistic infections used to confirm a diagnosis of AIDS. Any male under the age of 65 who develops EKS is considered to be terminally ill. In fact, after a diagnosis of EKS, the prognosis for life is generally not longer than 16 to 24 months. A young man diagnosed with Kaposi's sarcoma can be said to be terminally ill, whereas this cannot be said of an older man of 65 years or more.

The key factor that determines if a person is terminally ill is the judgment that the time of death is near. "Terminal refers to the endpoint when, regardless of the status of treatment, the patient's death is imminent."[19] Imminent generally means a prognosis of six months or less. Perhaps it is better to say that death is imminent when the progressive nature of the disease and the general condition of the person are such that death is more likely to be as a result of the disease or some complication inherent in the disease process than from some other factor. One can be said to be terminally ill, therefore, when one has a disease that, by its nature, is terminal, and when one is more likely to die of the effects of this illness than some other cause. This understanding of terminal illness will be important not only for determining the appropriateness of palliative care, but also in discussions of the cause of death in situations where treatment is withheld or withdrawn.

Symptom Control

Symptom control refers to the implementation of those measures, whether pharmacological, psychological, or spiritual, that keep the patient at an optimal level of functioning during the time remaining for that person.

When one is terminally ill, one has time. There may not be a lot of time, but some time does exist that can be put to use or wasted. In some instances, the quality of this time is lost by healthcare professionals who wait too long to admit that the person is terminally ill. Parkes writes:

> *It is clearly imperative for us, the care-givers, to try to help patient and family to make the best use of the time that remains to them. This is the main aim of terminal care and the most important single service we offer.*[20]

To achieve this aim, the measure by which all decisions should be made concerning the initiation of any clinical investigation or treatment of symptoms is whether or not the particular action being considered will result in an immediate and significantly improved quality of life.

The introduction of investigative procedures to determine the cause or causes behind the symptom is a debated issue in the care of the terminally ill. Some clinicians argue that terminally ill patients should be treated on a purely symptomatic basis regardless of the underlying cause of that symptom. The reasoning is that access to a laboratory or to radiological facilities, as well as the procedure itself, may prove too difficult for the person in the final days of life. On the other hand, if the clinician knows why a patient develops a particular symptom, it can be more effectively treated and its recurrence prevented. In any case, investigative procedures should never be used as grounds for delaying symptomatic treatment, and the investigation should always be directed specifically toward a particular symptom. Insofar as it is possible, it should be determined if the symptom experienced is the result of the progress of the malignant disease or if it arises from some unrelated development. Coincidental "sinister symptoms" are sometimes simpler to treat, and an accurate history and general physical examination may be sufficient.[21] At other times, additional simple investigative procedures, such as blood work or a computed tomography (CT) scan, may be required.

Investigations intended to characterize infections are generally beneficial to a patient. If the infection is asymptomatic, no investigation is required. Infections with severe symptoms, however, should be characterized and treated with appropriate antibiotics. The person will be more comfortable, and it is unlikely that the treatment of any serious intercurrent infection will significantly prolong life. Major infections occurring as an obvious part of the terminal event require no investigation and should be treated symptomatically.

Another investigation that may be appropriate would be to obtain a hemoglobin estimation. Cases of breathlessness, weakness, and fatigue in some severely anemic patients may be relieved by a blood transfusion. The relief is transitory but may be suitable for some at a particular time in the illness. The basic rule governing investigative procedures is whether the difficulty of the investigation and the discomfort brought to the person are outweighed by the measure of relief that can be expected if the symptom is treated in its cause rather than symptomatically.

As with investigation procedures, if a treatment will induce side effects that cause irritation, the person may be unable to enjoy or profit by it. Further, poorly administered treatment may not lengthen time at all but, in fact, shorten it. Poorly administered analgesics can take time away by causing debilitating somnolence or keeping the patient in such fear of recurring pain that he/she is too distracted to use pain-free time effectively.

Symptoms play different roles in different healthcare settings. In acute care, symptoms are guides to an understanding and correct diagnosis of the underlying illness. Once a diagnosis is made, medical treatment is directed toward the disease—the cause of the symptoms—not toward the symptoms themselves. In fact, too much attention directed toward the symptoms can undermine care by overlooking the treatable basis of the difficulty. In most cases of chronic care, symptomatic care is essential to improve the quality of the patient's life. In this instance, all symptoms are vigorously treated as they present themselves.

In palliative care, symptoms are viewed somewhat differently. Unlike acute care where the goal is a cure, the underlying cause of the symptom may not be treated. As already noted, treating the underlying cause may bring about more discomfort in the short term when the short term is all there is. Unlike chronic care, not all symptoms will be treated with the same vigor. The degree to which one goes to relieve a symptom and ensure that it does not return is greatly influenced by the shortness of time one has. Instead, a balance is sought between the potential immediate gain for the person and the overall cost in terms of side effects and energy expenditure. This balance can be discovered through an attempt to quantify the symptoms.

Although difficult and subjective, quantifying symptoms is helpful. The person is asked to specify any pain or discomfort experienced as being mild, moderate, or severe, rather than merely indicating pain in general. Further, general activity is assessed with factors that limit activity, such as pain or breathlessness, being carefully noted. How the patient passes the day, that is, in bed, working with his/her hands, or reading, as well as how much help is needed in these activities, is also documented. Such information adds little to the clinical assessment, but it is useful in evaluating the possible quality benefits of treatment.

All symptoms experienced by the person should be analyzed in some way. This is done either through a superficial or more thorough investigation. Treatment should consist of correcting the wrong or, if that is not appropriate, in relieving the symptoms. Patients dying with progressive diseases experience many symptoms, and good terminal care requires attention to all these simultaneously. Again, the underlying principle will be whether the treatment will allow the patient optimal functioning and significantly improve the quality of life.[22]

PRINCIPAL (CURATIVE) THERAPIES SEEN IN PALLIATIVE CARE

Cancer[23]

Surgery. Aggressive surgery. When a tumor is operable, surgery is the principal curative modality of cancer therapy.[24] The aim of surgery is the removal, or resection, of the primary tumor as well as a defined area surrounding the tumor to offer the best chance of avoiding local recurrence.[25] Regional lymph nodes may also be removed to prevent metastatic spread if there has been any infiltration by the tumor cells. This procedure is referred to as a *curative resection.*

In the past, such resections were believed to be most effective when most radical, that is, when as much tissue as possible surrounding the primary tumor was removed. The rationale behind such radical procedures was founded in the high incidence of local failure, a problem that remains even today.[26] In the last 10 years, however, there has been a movement toward less radical surgery. This has been made possible through a better appreciation of sophisticated disease staging, the emergence of new surgical procedures, as well as the combined use of surgery with other modalities such as radiation and chemotherapy. Today, curative resections are performed according to the basic principle that excision of the primary cancer should be made without going beyond the boundaries of the tissue or nodes infiltrated by the tumor.

Surgery may be appropriate in some cases of local recurrence. These include recurrence in instances of cancer of the mouth, after radiation in instances of cancer of the head and neck, or in cases of cervical cancer.[27] At times, there may be a recurrence associated with a different isolated tumor, not indicating the presence of disseminated disease. This is sometimes the case in instances of recurrent cancer of the stomach or colon. Surgical removal of the tumor is often the most effective therapy.

What might be called "second look" operations can also be employed as an extension of an aggressive approach to local recurrence. These exploratory procedures, which are performed without any clinically apparent recurrence, may be justified in cases where there has been frequent and isolated local recurrences not accompanied by metastases. In

101

these instances, any recurrence can be surgically removed with a reasonable chance of cure.

Surgery in cancer care is also used for the purpose of staging the cancer accurately. For example, a staging laparotomy in the case of Hodgkin's disease is helpful in determining whether radical radiation therapy or prolonged chemotherapy will be the most effective mode of treatment. Surgery may also be performed in conjunction with other therapies. For example, a pump oxygenator may be used to perfuse surgically isolated blood vessels in a limb, enabling hyperthermia, or to allow chemotherapy administration to be localized, thus protecting the body in general from harmful side effects. Both these innovations are relatively new to cancer therapy and will require more investigation before their usefulness is proved.[28]

Palliative surgery. When the prospect of cure exists, many demands can be reasonably made on the person with respect to pain, discomfort, and time. These might include extensive surgery to remove tumor masses or amputations. Even with the addition of extensive radiation or chemotherapy, these demands are generally seen as being worthwhile in view of an expected cure or remission. When the prospect of cure is diminished or becomes unrealistic, these demands become less tolerable, or even intolerable. In such instances, however, surgery may still be a viable therapy for palliation.

As an example, tumors that were first thought to be operative may be discovered to be inoperable during surgery. This may be caused by some direct extension to an adjacent vital organ. This would make the cancer incurable yet still resectable. This type of surgical intervention is known as a *palliative resection,* indicating that some of the cancer remains after the surgery. This type of palliative resection can provide a great deal of relief to the patient by preventing future symptoms. For example, an abdominoperineal resection could be performed even when there are some metastases to the liver. Although the surgery will not affect the overall prognosis of the person because of the cancerous liver, the person's quality of life will be heightened through the prevention of disabling tenesmus. In another example, bypass surgery of an obstructing esophageal carcinoma will not change the course of the progressive disease, but it will enable the person to swallow again.

When cure is no longer a reasonable goal, all surgery must be evaluated to determine if it will help secure a high quality of life with a minimal sacrifice. This sacrifice includes not only pain and discomfort, but also loss of independence and dignity, clouding of consciousness, and loss of time. For anyone who has a home, each day spent in the hospital, even the best hospital, generally is seen as a day wasted. Insofar as is possible, surgery in palliation ought to be directed toward the prevention of any future difficulties anticipated after an assessment of the patient's symptoms in light of the history of the disease. Once such an assessment is made, a program can be devised to relieve present symptoms and prevent further distress.

Symptoms that no one should have to endure for any period include intestinal colic, protracted vomiting,[29] inability to swallow one's own saliva, the stench of secondarily infected fungating tumors, the intractable itch of unrelieved obstructive jaundice, fecal or urinary incontinence, and the throbbing pain of pus under tension.[30] These must be controlled and often can be through the use of radiation or chemotherapy. When these fail, control can sometimes be achieved through the use of drug therapy, even if such use somewhat shortens the person's life. However, because of difficulties in drug metabolism arising from the patient's age, deteriorating condition, or the interaction of the several drugs being administered, this may not always be possible without affecting the person's awareness. This would deprive the person of valuable relationships, the opportunity to exercise personal independence, or the chance to live outside the hospital. In these instances, surgery can sometimes offer greater relief with less personal sacrifice.

Concerning the appropriateness of surgery relative to the sacrifice of the time investment involved, Williams writes:

> *Apart from minor procedures such as draining abscesses which are justifiable in the last days, my own rule of thumb is that one week spent in a surgical ward is justifiable if there is a prospect of three months' useful life at home, two weeks for six month's respite, while three weeks in a hospital is justified for a year of worthwhile survival.*[31]

In summary, surgery has a proper place not only in curative cancer therapy, but in palliative therapy as well. Palliative surgery is most appropriate when it anticipates and seeks to prevent difficulties that are expected to develop as the disease progresses. Surgery is still a possible option in the last few months of life when it can offer a greater benefit with fewer side effects than offered by other modalities. Perhaps the greatest factor in determining the sacrifice involved in surgery is that of time. Surgery seems justified as palliative when it can greatly enhance the time left, which itself is significantly greater than that required for the surgery and recovery.

Radiation Therapy. Radiation therapy involves the use of various forms of ionizing radiation in the treatment of disease. It is used largely, although not exclusively, for the management of malignant tumors. In this context, it is known as *beam irradiation.*[32] The goal of radiation is to kill cancerous cells with the hope of destroying, or at least reducing, a tumor. Since its introduction into medical practice with cobalt-60 25 years ago, there has been a steady increase in the success rate of controlling cancers treated primarily with radiation.

Today there are two types of radiation: orthovoltage, delivering energies of 200- to 300-kilovolt peak, and megavoltage, with energies above 1,000-kilovolt peak. An important distinction between these two types of radiation is that megavoltage does not deliver its maximum doses on the surface of the skin, as does orthovoltage. Instead, it reaches its peak at a depth of several millimeters to several centimeters. Depending on the total energy dosage, the skin may receive only 30 percent of the maximum dose, thus sparing a great deal of damage to healthy tissues.[33]

The radiation output of most accelerators is in the form of x-ray photons, although high-energy electrons are also used. Electrons are often advantageous because they have a definite range of penetration of tissue and are helpful in protecting sensitive tissue behind a tumor. Unfortunately, the maximum dose on the surface of the skin delivered by megavoltage is increased with the use of electron radiation. Although tissues deep behind the tumor may be spared, the skin surface in front of the tumor will suffer greater damage than it would with the use of photons. In situations where surface area and tissues behind the tumor need to be protected, a combination therapy of photons and electrons is often used.

Current therapy also includes the use of intracavity implants for tumor management. Under general anesthesia, an applicator is implanted in the person and loaded with a radioisotope source. This applicator can be easily removed or replaced at any time if necessary. These radioisotopes can also be implanted directly into the tumor and adjacent tissues. Ultimately, a combination of beam irradiation and intracavity or interstitial radioisotope therapy seems to offer the best means of achieving local tumor control with the lowest incidence of complications.

In cancer management, radiation has two broad aspects of usage. The first is known as *radical radiation,* the purpose of which is control of the tumor and the adjacent tissues and nodes. The second, *palliative radiation,* deals with tumors that have disseminated beyond the region of the primary tumor in an attempt to bring about symptomatic relief. These two types must always be distinguished at the beginning of therapy, since the cost to the patient in terms of time, money, and treatment-related complications will be substantially different. What may be justified in an attempt to cure may not be justified in an attempt to palliate.

Radical radiation. The appropriate use of radical radiation is determined by several factors. The theory that a given dose of radiation will destroy a certain type of cancer is no longer considered valid. Instead, it appears that the *size* of the tumor to be treated, not the *type* of tumor, must be considered in determining the appropriate quantity of radiation required to kill the entire cell population of the tumor. Other factors involved include the growth rate, the pattern of growth, and the vascularity of the tumor.[34]

The dose at which the radiation can be delivered is limited by the tolerance of the surrounding normal tissue. Injury to other tissues and organs may represent a significant risk because the difference between doses required for the control of the tumor and those causing significant complications is quite small. Fig. 4.2 shows the probability of control and complications plotted together.[35] The separation of the curves gives a clear indication of the potential for therapeutic gain while, at the same time, indicating that any small increase in dose will not only result in an increase of control, but will also bring about a substantial increase in the risk of complications:

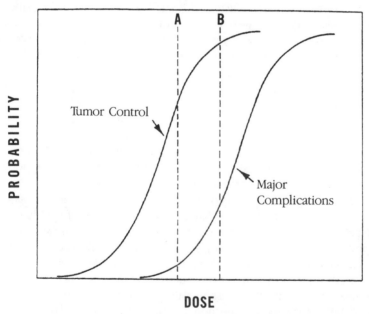

Fig. 4.2 Probability of Tumor Control and Complications
Plotted Against Radiation Dosage

The type and severity of the complications depend on many factors, such as the size of the tumor treated, the area treated, and so forth. Whether or not these side effects are acceptable will always be determined in light of the requirements for and the possibility of a cure.

A complication known as "dry mouth" can result from radiation directed toward the salivary gland in treating an oral cancer. Sterilization is a complication that can result from radiation to the pelvic region. A feared complication is the radiation causing a cancer. Although radiation exposure is known to have a possible carcinogenic effect, tumors induced in adults who have received therapeutic radiation with modern techniques are uncommon.

In many instances, radiation therapy is considered to be preferable to other modalities. It is a valuable alternative to surgery in cases of early-stage carcinoma of the cervix; early carcinoma of the larynx, breast, and prostate; as well as with most skin cancers. Radiation therapy is also more useful than surgery in cases of Hodgkin's disease and malignant lymphomas, oat cell carcinoma of the lung, and advanced-stage carcinoma of the cervix and prostate.

The choice of radiation over surgery may also be made in consideration of factors other than effectiveness, such as functional and cosmetic considerations. With laryngeal cancer, radiation may be preferable to surgery because it will preserve an essentially normal voice. On the other hand, a young woman with early-stage carcinoma of the cervix may wish to remain fertile and choose surgery.

In general, although surgery is good for macroscopic tumors that are clinically identifiable, it is generally less effective in cases of a microscopic spread in the area of the tumor. Similarly, radiation will probably be ineffective in dealing with a large tumor mass, yet be used with success for isolated cells and microscopic tumors. A combination of the two therapeutic approaches appears to offer the best chances of tumor management. Today, preoperative and postoperative radiation are often employed.

Palliative radiation. Once it has been determined that cure is no longer a reasonable goal, radiation may still be a valuable therapy for palliation. Unlike palliative surgery, which is most often used to anticipate symptoms or to prolong life, palliative radiation seeks primarily to alleviate distressing symptoms as quickly as possible. Preventive radiation most often imposes a burden on the patient in terms of time, effort, and money, which may never be balanced by benefits.[36] Success in palliation depends primarily on the extent of the disease and the functional status of the patient. The patient's previous treatments may also be a factor. For example, radiation of extensive amounts of bone marrow to relieve multiple bone metastases is not possible in a patient whose white blood cell count is below normal because of prior extensive use of chemotherapy or radiation.[37]

The use of radiation for palliation is determined by the limited expectation of life and the need to avoid additional discomfort. The radiologist must be able to make a correct assessment of the situation with a minimum of time-consuming investigation to determine what can be reasonably hoped for and what is impossible. Some factors that influence the potential value of radiation are the radiosensitivity of the tumor,[38] the radiotolerance of the surrounding tissue,[39] and the degree to which the tumor and the normal tissues have been irradiated in the past.[40] Other considerations include the availability of facilities and trained personnel, the overall time required for the patient to receive the therapy, technical radiation factors such as total dose, treatment volume and energy of radiation (orthovoltage or megavoltage), and the overall management of the patient's needs as opposed to the resolution of a single problem.

This last consideration, the patient's overall comfort, is of particular importance. Radiation can be harmful in the long term even if it is palliative in the short term. This is particularly true when a tumor is infiltrating a neighboring organ such as the bladder or bowel. In these instances, radiation, even in small doses, may lead to fistula formation. In this case, the symptoms that result will be more distressing than those of the untreated tumor. Further, it is generally not considered wise to direct radiation toward the pelvis of a patient dying with uremia associated with advanced pelvic cancer. The relief of the ureteric obstruction may keep the patient alive just long enough to develop more distressing terminal symptoms, such as severe pelvic pain or, in the case of a woman, an offensive vaginal discharge.[41]

When palliative radiation is considered appropriate, it should be given without delay and without numerous visits to the radiologist. Effective palliation is sometimes achieved in a single visit, but more generally a course of five to six treatments over two to three weeks is necessary.[42] Daily treatments over several weeks are generally not considered to be appropriate. The aim is to relieve symptoms with the lowest possible dose in the fewest possible treatments. Side effects at this stage of the disease are few, and it is important not to confuse the effects of the therapy with those of the progressive disease. The benefits of the therapy must be weighed against the price paid in terms of time and trouble. Two common difficulties that lend themselves to palliative radiation and worthy of note here because of their importance in overall cancer management are metastatic bone pain and brain metastases.

Metastatic bone pain is the palliative situation seen most frequently by radiation therapists. Primary tumors of the lung, breast, or prostate comprise the majority of these cases.[43] Richter reports that 70 percent of those treated with palliative radiation will receive some relief within four weeks following therapy. A study at the Veterans' Hospital in Philadelphia reported that almost all patients showed improvement by the second week of therapy, and most were completely free of pain by the fourth week. This period of relief was generally longer than the median survival time of five months.[44]

Metastases to the brain, often the most feared consequence of cancer, require proper treatment. Seizures and headaches resulting from increased cranial pressure can be significantly relieved by palliative cranial radiation given at different treatment schedules. Richter reports a positive response rate of 60 percent, with an average survival time of four to six months.[45]

Chemotherapy. Aggressive chemotherapy. Chemotherapy, the use of various chemicals to control a disease, is associated with a history of negative side effects ranging from hair loss and nausea to vomiting and a general physical deterioration. Some of this association is the result of unrealistic expectations of what the therapy could do as well as its poor administration.[46] Although much of this negative publicity remains today, there are 35 clinically useful chemotherapeutic agents, making chemotherapy one of the major modalities of treatment for a number of cancers. Chemotherapy can offer long-term control for such cancers as acute leukemia in children, Hodgkin's disease, testicular cancer, breast cancer, and a number of soft tissue and bone sarcomas. For this reason, in spite of the fact that alone it is rarely curative, chemotherapy belongs in the aggressive phase of the treatment of malignant diseases.[47] The use of chemotherapy, however, is a cautious affair. The total extent of the disease should be known and proved to be malignant before it is initiated.[48]

Most tumors are not detectable until they are between 0.5 and 1.0 cm in diameter. At this stage, the tumor will already have undergone 26 to 30 cell divisions, growing to a total of approximately one billion cells. This growth can take place over the span of seven years.[49] During this time, it is possible that one or several metastases will have already occurred. When this happens, the total number of tumor cells throughout the body will far exceed the clinically apparent disease. Undetected and untreated, these metastases could develop into a clinically evident metastatic cancer of more than one trillion cells per mass.[50] The value of chemotherapy lies in its ability to control these occult metastases. The advantages of treating the metastases before they become clinically apparent are obvious.

Chemotherapy achieves its effect by poisoning the cancerous cells with which it comes in contact. It is possible that chemotherapy reduces the number of tumor cells to a small critical level, at which point the person's immune system can finish the task of eliminating the cancerous cells.

It has been found that an effective dose of medication will kill a fixed *percentage* of the tumor cells present, not a fixed *number*. This is true regardless of how many cells are present at the time the therapy is initiated. It is necessary, therefore, to administer the chemotherapy in cycles to achieve the maximum effect. The therapy is administered in a given amount, x number of times for x number of days.

The cycles in which the therapy is administered involve periods when the therapy is stopped. This is necessary because the chemotherapy affects normal as well as cancerous cell growth. Therapy must allow periods of rest long enough to give the healthy cells the opportunity to heal without allowing the cancer cells to regenerate.

Toxicity must also be accounted for in this cycle. Some agents have an affinity to particular cells in the body. For example, adriamycin has an affinity to cardiac cells, resulting in cardiogenic toxicity. The cancer may be controlled, but the person could be left with severe heart disease. The possible toxic effects to the person need to be accurately predicted so that supportive therapy can be administered. For example, granulocyte transfusions can be administered to help control problems of anemia, bleeding, and infection, which can pose major complications in the administration of chemotherapy.

Difficulties in the use of chemotherapy for tumor management arise from the complicated mechanism of tumor growth. Tumors develop in cycles. At any given time in the tumor's development, only a proportion of the cells will be actively dividing. This is known as the *growth fraction*.[51] In the early stages of the tumor, most of the cancerous cells are dividing. As the tumor grows, however, more and more of the cells become inactive. The exact duration of each phase is not known for each tumor, although it is known that the inactive phase can be very long.

Most chemotherapeutic agents are effective only against cells during some phase of division. Some "cycle-specific" agents are more effective against dividing cells than inactive cells. Other "phase-specific" agents are only effective during a specific phase of the cell cycle, such as during mitosis. A third group, "cycle-phase nonspecific" agents, act equally against dividing and inactive cells. Because little is known about the growth fractions of specific tumors, the choice of a chemotherapeutic agent in particular instances is very difficult to make. Some attempts have been made to stimulate cell division and thereby make tumors more sensitive to cycle-specific and phase-specific agents, but these have been unsuccessful.[52]

In the administration of chemotherapeutic agents, animal studies had suggested that the intermittent use of high doses of phase-specific or cycle-specific agents were more effective than the continuous use of low doses. However, this has not proved to be clinically true for human beings in all cases. Although this regimen is successful against human tumors with rapid cell division such as Hodgkin's disease and diffuse forms of non-Hodgkin's lymphomas, the principle does not hold for tumors with slow cell division such as cancers of the lung, colon, and breast. In the latter cases, continuous low doses have proved to be more effective.

In the early days of chemotherapy, an agent was selected for use based on the predicted effect of the drug shown in experimentation. If a clinical response occurred with this agent, it was usually for a limited time. When no further response was detected, another single agent was used. This second agent generally gave a response of a shorter duration than that of the first. This regimen of using successive single agents was continued until no further response was obtained. Later, a principle was borrowed from the treatment of general bacteria. It was known that some bacteria could remain immune to treatment if a resistance could be built up. This resistance was made possible when medication was administered in a step-by-step progression, or if the bacteria were associated with some organisms inherently resistant to the drug being used. If the same were true of cancerous cells, then multiple agents with different mechanisms of action could improve the response rate and duration.

This theory was first applied to hematological malignancies and met with great success. Since then, numerous combinations have been tried against all tumors. Today different combinations of chemotherapeutic agents are used based on the following criteria:

1. Each agent in the combination should be active against a given tumor alone. Ineffective single agents do not become effective when used in combination.
2. Agents should have different mechanisms of action. Duplicating mechanisms does not enhance the effectiveness.
3. The toxic effects of the agents should not overlap in order that each drug can be given at the near maximum tolerated doses. Agents have different as well as similar toxicities; thus they can be combined to maximize effect without adding significantly to the overall toxicity of the therapy.[53]

Palliative chemotherapy. The use of chemotherapeutic agents with the terminally ill is limited. Most chemotherapeutic agents have unpleasant side effects, and the response to treatment can be delayed by as much as four to six weeks.[54] In addition, the palliative value of chemotherapy is not as predictable as other therapies such as radiation.

A successful response to these drugs is usually associated with a prolonging of life.[55] Glick reports that patients who show some response to chemotherapy, even with disseminated metastatic disease, generally feel better and live longer than those who show no response.[56] It seems, then, that the use of chemotherapy has more to do with prolonging of life for some, rather than with symptom control and a raised quality of life for terminally ill persons in general. It has already been pointed out that the mere prolonging of life is not the proper goal of palliative care as defined here with regard to care for the terminally ill person. Its use, therefore, is restricted.

When deemed appropriate, chemotherapy for the terminally ill person is best administered orally, since this requires a minimum of supervision and monitoring with fewer and more controllable side effects. In these instances, the administration of a single agent is generally preferred. Although single agents tend to be less effective, they are more easily administered and often have fewer toxic side effects. For example, in a case of breast cancer, 100 mg of cyclophosphamide taken orally on a daily basis may give some temporary benefit without the side effects of nausea, bone marrow depression, or hair loss. Bladder irritation can be avoided if the drug is taken in the morning with plenty of fluids throughout the day. The intravenous administration of adriamycin, the most effective single agent with breast cancer, is associated with such a high incidence of balding that its use with the terminally ill patient is generally considered inappropriate.

Most people who receive care during the end stages of a progressive, terminal disease have already made a decision that aggressive therapy in the use of chemotherapeutic agents is no longer appropriate. The discontinuation of these agents is made easier when other symptoms are controlled and the person is already comfortable. There may be a place for continuing low dosages of these agents, even when there is little chance of affecting the disease process, if the patient believes these are beneficial.[57] It is not always easy to know whether the drug is responsible for an apparently static state in the course of the disease. Drugs may be inappropriate at one moment, but, if the patient's general condition should improve and a longer prognosis is evident, they might become appropriate to assist some natural remission.

Circumstances in which some type of chemotherapy might be appropriate for terminal, palliative care seem to be few. One possible case might be with ovarian carcinoma. If chemotherapy was not part of aggressive therapy, it could be considered in palliative care, especially when there is the frequent need to tap an accumulation of fluids in the abdominal cavity. Cases of cervical cancer require the use of highly toxic agents such as adriamycin and methotrexate and therefore are not usually considered. Other cases, such as gastrointestinal and bronchial cancer, are better controlled by radiation than chemotherapy.

People with lymphoproliferative disorders and leukemias constitute special cases in terminal care. Patients with these malignancies have been treated previously with chemotherapeutic agents and usually with blood or blood products over such an extended period that they often come to be viewed almost as a way of life. This makes a decision to stop such treatment difficult. However, if symptom control is given greater emphasis as the disease progresses, a change in therapy away from these agents is possible.

It would seem, therefore, that the use of chemotherapeutic agents in the management of cancer has an important role to play in aggressive therapy, especially in the treatment of possible disseminated and metastatic tumors that are not clinically evident at the diagnosis. However, as the disease process continues, their use is limited to those situations when the side effects of such agents are outweighed by the value of a prolonged life. When quality of life is of paramount importance, as with palliative care for the terminally ill person, chemotherapy seems to be of little real use unless the patient has some spontaneous remission.

AIDS

Prevention and Therapy. To date, there is no vaccine to prevent human immunodeficiency virus (HIV) infection, no proven medical therapy available to reverse the effect of infection on the immune system, and nothing to prevent the development of AIDS or AIDS-related complex (ARC). In developments leading to a possible vaccine, Zagury of the Pierre and Marie Curie University in Paris inoculated himself and 10 Zairian volunteers in 1987 with recombinant vaccinia virus containing a gene from the AIDS virus.[58] Vaccinia virus has been widely used to immunize people against smallpox. Zagury is testing a genetically engineered form of it containing a gene of the HTLV-III$_8$ isolate that forms the protein envelope of the virus. In Zagury's own words, however, "I do not have a vaccine for AIDS; I have a candidate vaccine."[59]

Reaction to Zagury's experiment has been mixed. Moss of the National Institute of Allergy and Infectious Diseases (NIAID), who supplied some materials used in the experiment, was quick to indicate that the materials were provided for experiments with animals, not human beings. This prototype vaccine has neither been approved nor even reviewed by the

Food and Drug Administration. Mayer and Opal report that "the prospects for a vaccine in the near future appear to be unlikely."[60]

Surgery. Robinson et al. concluded a study in 1987 that sought to determine what surgical procedures might be of benefit to patients with AIDS.[61] Their study consisted of 21 patients with an average age of 36 years at the time of surgery. Thirty-one surgical procedures were performed. Seven of these included such emergencies as thoracostomies, celiotomies, and one craniotomy. The other 21 were elective procedures done for diagnostic and therapeutic purposes.

In this study, the approximate average length of time the patients lived from the time AIDS was diagnosed until death was 31 weeks. The range was from 2 weeks to 14 months. For AIDS patients in general, this same period from diagnosis to death is estimated to be approximately 29 weeks.[62] Robinson et al. state that, although these calculations may be of no predictive value, they do allow a comparison. Surgery, when medically appropriate, may be of only minimal time value. The criteria of Williams cited earlier—that, apart from minor procedures, one week in the hospital for surgery is justifiable if there will be three months of enjoyment at home—would seem to minimize the value of surgery for the person dying with AIDS.[63]

Radiation therapy. The use of radiation therapy in cases of AIDS is associated with one of the most common malignancies associated with AIDS, Kaposi's sarcoma (KS). KS is the basis for the initial diagnosis of AIDS in 24 percent of all cases reported in the United States.[64] One study suggests that at least 33 percent of all cases of AIDS show some involvement of KS,[65] although it does seem more likely to develop in homosexually oriented men than in others. This is thought to be caused partly by the use of nitrate inhalants as a sexual stimulant.[66]

The incidence of KS among AIDS patients has presented some unique difficulties. Classic KS (CKS), found among men 65 years of age and older, is generally easier to manage than the form related to AIDS, epidemic KS (EKS). In cases of CKS, the lesions are highly radiosensitive and respond well to doses within the range of tolerance of surrounding tissue. Because of the noncritical location of the lesions, their relative indolence, and the age of the patient, relatively simple superficial therapy is generally all that is required.

This is not the case with EKS, in which there is generally a wide variety of sites involved. This, along with the wide disparity in the patient's health status, necessitates a much more carefully tailored radiation response. The lack of experience in treating EKS, identified only five years ago, has made the determination of this response difficult.

A study by Nobler et al. supports the notion that KS does respond promptly to radiation. This can be of a twofold benefit to the person. Any shrinkage of the lesions or a reduction in the edema will not only provide greater comfort, but may also help to eliminate some of the stigma of AIDS by making the lesions, which have come to be associated with AIDS, less visible. In addition, radiation is less likely than chemotherapy to further threaten the person's already depressed immune system. Malignant lymphomas are also sensitive to radiation. Local palliative radiation has often resulted in the complete disappearance of lymphomatous masses.

In another study, Cooper and Fried also found that radiation for palliation was generally successful.[67] This needs to be tempered, however, with the fact that, in EKS, a good response at one site does not mean that another site will respond as well. Also, by citing toxicity in some cases, Cooper and Fried came to conclusions that are a little more cautious than those put forth by Nobler et al.

Cooper and Fried focused primarily on the control of pain. Of the 43 patients in the study, 24 patients indicated that pain was a significant problem at a total of 26 different sites. Radiation led to complete relief in 14 sites, partial relief in 3, and no relief in 4. The pain was not able to be evaluated in 5 sites because two patients died shortly after treatment and 3 refused any follow-up. Patients in the study who received 10 fractions or more obtained relief anywhere from midway through the treatment to 20 weeks after treatment had begun. The average time was 7.5 weeks. Those patients who received a single fraction obtained relief in an average of 15 weeks. What is significant is that there were no recorded relapses of pain at any site that had been treated.

Cooper and Fried conclude that radiation therapy should be reserved for the palliation of EKS in those instances where one or more sites of disease are particularly painful or are interfering with normal function. Patients with widespread disease and no particular problem at any site should be dissuaded from treatment.

Nobler et al. made reference to the benefit of radiation in reducing the stigma often attached to KS: the presence of noticeable lesions that are not only unattractive, but in a young man, are also indicative of AIDS. Cooper and Fried suggest that, rather than the use of radiation, asymptomatic lesions ought to be covered with make-up to reduce their visibility. It should be noted that, even if bulky and disfiguring lesions are treated with radiation for cosmetic reasons, they tend to leave a residual pigmentation after they flatten. Patients should know before treatment begins that some form of make-up will still be required.

Chemotherapy. One chemotherapeutic agent currently being studied in the treatment of AIDS is Azidothymidine (AZT). AZT was first found to be an effective inhibitor of a C-type murine retrovirus replication in vitro more than 12 years ago. However, no application of the drug was found in medicine until testing began to determine its effect on HIV replication. A study conducted by Fischl et al.[68] has shown that AZT can decrease mortality and the frequency of opportunistic infections in a selected group of patients with AIDS or ARC. These conclusions have been supported by other studies, such as that reported at a 1987 conference of the National Institute of Health.[69]

There are serious side effects associated with the use of AZT. Richman et al. report that, although significant clinical benefit has been documented, serious adverse reactions, particularly bone marrow suppression, have also been observed. Nausea, insomnia, and severe headaches have also been associated with the use of AZT. Richman et al. conclude that:

Although a subset of patients tolerated AZT for an extended period with few toxic effects, the drug should be administered with caution because of its toxicity and the limited experience with it to date.[70]

Studies to test the usefulness of AZT to prevent AIDS or ARC in people who are asymptomatic HIV positive are being planned. The risks involved in the use of AZT, however, have made such efforts very controversial. The use of other antiretroviral chemotherapeutic agents, such as Ribavirin, are also being tested. The initial results of randomized, placebo-controlled tests indicate that selected antiretroviral chemotherapy will result in some clinical benefit to patients, including those with advanced disease. Although such agents as AZT do not represent a cure, they do represent the first step in developing a practical chemotherapy against HIV, as well as other human retroviruses.

Treatment of Opportunistic Infections. No discussion of AIDS would be complete without a discussion of the treatment of opportunistic infections.[71] These infections constitute the major life-threatening manifestation of the suppression of the immune system brought on by HIV infection and AIDS. The difficulties found in treating these infections, as with the difficulty in finding an effective way to prevent or eliminate the virus directly, give insight into the rationale of palliative care for AIDS patients.

According to the Centers for Disease Control (CDC), 63 percent of the first 16,500 people diagnosed with AIDS had *Pneumocystis carinii* pneumonia (PCP) at the time the diagnosis was made.[72] Kovacs reports, however, that the incidence of PCP, along with other statistics indicating the presence of infections, is understated.[73] Because these infections were recorded only at the time of diagnosis, they do not take into account infections that developed later. In fact, death with AIDS is directly attributable to infections such as PCP in more than 85 percent of the cases. Only 7 percent of the deaths reported have been shown to be related to malignancies such as KS.[74]

Given the lack of a vaccine or a cure, the need for effective diagnosis and treatment of opportunistic infections is paramount. Part of the difficulty in achieving this is rooted in a delay in diagnosis. This may result from subtle or nonspecific symptoms, particularly in an otherwise healthy person. Even when an accurate diagnosis of an infection is made, however, there are many management problems.

To date, there is no documented effective therapy available for many of the infections related to AIDS. This is true, for example, for the Epstein-Barr virus. In other instances where treatment is available, a high proportion of people with AIDS suffer from side effects not usually associated with those treatments.

Another difficulty is the high incidence of failure and relapse associated with virtually every opportunistic infection that can be successfully treated. PCP, for example, recurs in about 20 percent of those treated. Another infection, cryptococcosis, recurs in over 50 percent of those treated.[75] Although there are effective treatments available for the four infections most often associated with death in cases of AIDS, all these are associated with relatively high failure and relapse rates.

Most recently, neurological complications of an HIV infection have been reported. Barnes estimates that as many as one half to two thirds of the AIDS patients in the United States will develop moderate to severe neurological problems.[76] Clark and Vinters make reference to an "AIDS-dementia complex," characterized initially by an impaired memory and concentration, as well as some motor function difficulties such as the loss of muscle coordination, leg weakness, and tremors. Behavioral disturbances, such as apathy, withdrawal, and sometimes psychosis, have also been observed. The disease ultimately leaves the patient with severe dementia, incontinence, and an inability to speak or walk. Most often a CT scan indicates cortical atrophy.[77] Tuazon and Labriola suggest that until an effective antiretroviral agent or some other form of therapy is discovered, the management of AIDS patients will be mainly supportive in nature. Attempts should be made primarily to maintain motor activity in order to prevent loss of muscle tone and function.[78]

Palliative Care. What emerges from this brief overview of some of the treatments for HIV infection and the opportunistic infections associated with AIDS is a rationale for the emergence of palliative care. The absence of a vaccine, a cure, or a proven effective treatment for AIDS or for the opportunistic infections associated with it illustrates the importance of palliative care in the care of people with AIDS. When a cure is not possible, a person can still be assisted in the task of becoming well.

The condition of AIDS has been referred to as the terminal event of the HIV infection and disease process. Given the reality that a cure is not possible, the most anyone can hope for medically is effective management of the disease. This can only be accomplished with difficulty. Just as the total mass of tumor present in the advanced clinical phase of cancer patients gives insight into the failure of conventional therapy to control the disease process adequately, so does the incidence of failure, severe side effects, and relapse regarding the treatment of opportunistic infections give insight into the inability of medicine, at present, to manage adequately this disease process. When this is the case, the appropriateness of palliative care emerges as the person seeks to put some order and meaning into what is happening.

The medical reality is that the person cannot hope to be healthy again. The statistics surrounding treatment indicate that the time may come when the person will choose not to treat yet another infection. At that time, perhaps more than at any other, the person will want care that has as its primary goal the well-being of the person, who happens to be dying with AIDS.

PAIN MANAGEMENT

Pain is an important physiological mechanism. Among its positive aspects are its ability to warn of danger, increase anxiety levels to mobilize coping mechanisms, seek to limit injury by provoking an immediate response, limit activity of the injured part to promote healing, and teach an aversion to potentially harmful stimuli.[79]

The role pain plays in ensuring survival is attested to by injuries suffered by those who have lost their sense of pain, such as lepers. Cousins writes that the loss of fingers, toes, and the like is associated with a lack of knowledge that an injury is taking place during the performance of ordinary tasks because a sense of pain is lacking. Eye trouble can sometimes be the result of the inability of the eye to become irritated by dirt, thus not triggering the natural eyewash of blinking.[80] Writing about Paul Brands, a physician working with lepers in Vellore, India, Cousins comments:

> *He is a doctor who, if he could, would move heaven and earth just to return the gift of pain to people who do not have it. For pain is*

*both the warning system and the protective mechanism that
enables the individual to defend the integrity of his body. Its signals
may not always be readily intelligible, but at least they are there,
and the individual can mobilize his response.*[81]

Regardless of the positive attributes of pain, it is nevertheless feared and generally avoided at all costs. With cancer, pain is of the greatest concern. In fact, cancer is often understood as being synonymous with pain.[82] It is no wonder that, more than death, people with a terminal illness fear the process of dying. They are afraid of dying in pain.

The term *cancer* does not necessarily imply, and need not be equated with, pain. Pain is usually not present during the early phases of the disease process, and as many as 50 percent of patients with advanced cancer experience no pain or only negligible discomfort. It is estimated that another 10 percent experience only mild to moderate pain. The remaining 40 percent experience severe, intractable pain[83] that, although more difficult, can be controlled. The necessary medical, pharmacological, surgical, psychosocial, radiological, and physical interventions do exist to control cancer pain and to help people cope with the disease and its symptoms.[84]

The identification of cancer with pain remains, however, because optimal use of these interventions is often not made in acute care settings. In acute care, patients generally need to ask for an analgesic as they watch the clock indicate how much longer they must wait, or they are so heavily medicated that any meaningful communication with others is eliminated. Sometimes the medication may be allowed to reach toxic levels, resulting in further complications in the person's condition.

The loss of an appreciation for the benefits that the experience of pain may have for the individual may be rooted in a misunderstanding of pain. Medicine's apparent inability to control it, which further detracts from a positive evaluation of pain, may also be rooted in its misunderstanding.[85] This misunderstanding flows from the fact that pain has not been adequately defined. The *Taber's Cyclopedic Medical Dictionary,* for example, defines pain as "a sensation in which a person experiences discomfort, distress, or suffering due to irritation of or stimulation of sensory nerves, especially pain sensors."[86] As a definition, it is too ambiguous and too general to be of much clinical value.

A more useful definition, the one that will be used here, is one offered by Benoliel et al. She defines pain as (1) a personal, private sensation of hurt, (2) a harmful stimulus that signals current or impending tissue damage, and (3) a pattern of responses that operate to protect the organism from harm.[87] Using this definition as an outline can highlight some of the key issues in appropriate pain management.

Definition of Pain

Personal, Private Sensation of Hurt. It is not possible for one person to really know what it is like for another to be in pain. Although everyone knows the experience of pain, each person knows the experience of his/her "own" pain, not the experience of another's. Pain is highly personal. How pain is experienced is greatly determined by the meaning that a person gives to that pain, the way the individual defines his/her life situation, and the individual's past experiences. For some people, pain is not experienced as being negative or evil. These people have somehow placed so much spiritual significance in the experience that they simply "offer it up" and move on. Other people have life styles that are in such a state of confusion and anxiety that the slightest pinprick is a major tragedy. Still others, remembering a previously painful experience at the dentist, begin to feel pain as soon as they are seated in the chair, even before the dentist has entered the room.

Cultural differences will also affect a person's attitude toward, and experience of, pain. Although some cultures seek to avoid pain at almost any cost, such as here in the United States, other cultures prize the ability to endure great suffering as evidence of maturity and integrity. One's sex can also be a factor in determining how a person ought to respond to the experience of pain. In the United States, young girls may be allowed to cry as they please, whereas at the same time and even in the same experience, young boys might be told that they should not cry. A society's attitudes toward pain and gender can almost dictate how a person is to respond, regardless of the pain experienced.

Another factor in the experience of pain will be the time duration. This will be seen in more detail below, but it is important to note here because the time factor affects the person psychologically. If the person expects the pain to pass within a short time, he/she will be better able to deal with it than when the pain is protracted over an extended period. The longer one experiences pain, the more intense that experience becomes. The experience may become still worse if hope of relief fades.

This personal dimension of the experience of pain is based on the premise that one's cognitive and emotional reactions can influence the perception of that experience.[88] This is supported by the observation that physical tissue damage alone cannot always account for the degree of pain experienced.[89] Studies further support this premise, showing that, although pain is determined primarily by the disease, it is also profoundly influenced by psychological factors such as the person's past life, religious beliefs, anxiety about the welfare of loved ones, and feelings of guilt that often arise in attempts to find some meaning in the experience.[90] Fears of progressive loss of bodily function and abandonment by others will also affect the perception of one's pain.

Twycross has shown that an individual's pain threshold, the level at which the individual will begin to experience intolerable levels of discomfort, can vary according to psychological as well as physical factors. These are shown in Table 4.1.[91]

Table 4.1 Factors that Modify Pain Threshold

Discomfort		Relief of symptoms	
Insomnia		Sleep	
Fatigue		Rest	
Anxiety		Sympathy	
Fear		Understanding	
Anger	THRESHOLD	Diversion	THRESHOLD
Sadness	LOWERED	Elevation of mood	RAISED
Depression			
Mental isolation		Analgesics	
Introversion		Anxiolytics	
(Past experience)		Antidepressants	

Adapted from Robert G. Twycross, "Relief of Pain," in *The Management of Terminal Disease,* ed. Cicely M. Saunders, Edward Arnold Publishers Ltd., London, 1978, p. 68.

It should be noted in Table 4.1 that the threshold can be modified in either direction, increasing or decreasing the pain experience. This suggests that pain control has to do with more than merely the administration of analgesics. Because pain is a personal experience, its relief requires "personal" and not merely "drug" intervention. Although drug therapy is one of the major modalities for pain relief, it is only one of many. Analgesics are most effective when combined with other, personal modalities. Lipman has concluded that neither the best drug therapy without psychosocial support nor the most attentive loving without appropriate drug therapy will be effective for pain management.[92]

Harmful Stimulus that Signals Current or Impending Tissue Damage. There are two very different experiences of pain, differences that have not always been adequately appreciated.[93] These are the experiences of acute and chronic pain. These two types or components of pain are distinguished by different physiological processes involving two different groups of physiological systems; the lateral group and the medial group. Arising from different physiological groups, acute and chronic pain involve different experiences, each of which will involve its own appropriate response. Any understanding of palliative care, with its emphasis on symptom control, must entail a clear understanding of the symptoms of pain as it is experienced by the person.

Acute pain. Acute pain is experienced through the lateral physiological system. This lateral system is characterized by the speed and priority with which some stimulus is transmitted from the point of stimulation to the brainstem, where this information is processed.

The lateral system works by transmitting "phasic" information, which is brief and passing, from the point where the senses are alerted to the brainstem. The information moves quickly through the nervous system, taking priority over other messages that may be travelling the same route. This priority ensures that some response will be set in motion as quickly as possible. The information gained by the stimulus is instantly integrated with other bodily functions in order to initiate some immediate and appropriate physical response. Loscalzo suggests that the integration of the stimulus with motor systems is meant to trigger a "fight-or-flight response."[94] The purpose of the response is to minimize possible damage. A good example is the touching of a hot object. The stimulus triggers an instant response to move away from the object. The pain experienced is time limited, lessening over a relatively brief period. It is intended primarily to trigger a response that will cause the person to move quickly. Once that is accomplished, its usefulness passes.

Chronic pain. Chronic pain is associated with the more complex physiological mechanisms of the medial group. This group is characterized by a much slower transmitting of some stimulus and the frequent passing of the information concerning the stimulus from one neuron to another. This less specific relay of information from the point of stimulus to the brainstem results in its more general integration, and thus a less specific response. The result is a tonic or continuous pain. The message is intended to last for hours or even longer to indicate the presence of damage. The behavior triggered by this response is meant to be a limiting influence, limiting physical activity for the purpose of preventing reinjury and facilitating rest and healing.

The purpose of these two components of pain is clearly distinguished. Acute pain is rapid, intending to trigger an immediate response to limit damage. Chronic pain is slow and continuous, intending to limit activity so that damage already done can be repaired. These two purposes are achieved principally through the transient nature of the former and the persistent nature of the latter. It is these two natures, more than anything else, that distinguish the two different experiences of pain. Twycross points to this by referring to acute pain as an "event" and chronic pain as a "situation."[95] As an event, pain happens and passes. As a situation, it is impossible to predict when pain will end. Chronic pain usually gets worse rather than better, lacks positive meaning, and frequently expands to occupy the person's whole attention. When this happens, life itself may seem no longer worth living.

Management. The aim in both acute and chronic pain management is the same: to relieve the pain. However, given the differences between the two components of pain, how this is done will be different. Acute pain can be controlled more easily because the person knows, intellectually at least, that it is going to pass. It becomes easier to wait for medication, and PRN (*pro re nata,* as required) orders seem appropriate because eventually the medication is not going to be required. Chronic pain, on the other hand, is not going to go away, and there is little, if any, hope that further medication will not be needed on a regular basis. Medication "as required" does not work with chronic pain. It is always required. Further, pain is its own algesic; it makes itself worse.[96] Management in cases of chronic pain has to do not so much with relief as with prevention. Chronic pain control has to do with keeping pain from emerging in the first place, not in subduing it after it has surfaced. A comparison of the differences in the relief of acute and chronic pain is illustrated by Twycross in Table 4.2.[97]

Table 4.2 Comparison of Analgesic Use in Acute and Chronic Pain

	Acute	Chronic
Aim	Pain relief	Pain relief
Sedation	Often desirable	Usually undesirable
Desired duration of effect	2-4 hours	As long as possible
Timing	As required (on demand)	Regularly (in anticipation)
Dose	Usually standard	Individually determined
Route	Injection	By mouth
Adjuvant medication	Uncommon	Common

Adapted from Robert G. Twycross, "Relief of Pain," in *The Management of Terminal Disease,* ed. Cicely M. Saunders, Edward Arnold Publishers Ltd., London, 1978, p. 72.

Acute pain is often described as being mild, moderate, or severe. Because of the long-lasting nature of chronic pain, it is more difficult to describe. As the person becomes exhausted from lack of sleep caused by pain, the pain will seem much worse even if physiologically it should be lessened. As shown in Fig. 4.3, Lipman describes chronic pain as moving in a circular continuum from aching to agony.[98]

Fig. 4.3 Chronic Pain: Aching to Agony

The objective in treatment is to move away from agony to the aching, a situation most people can tolerate. The shift is possible in part by treatment that addresses what Lipman calls the three dimensions of chronic pain: the physical, the psychological, and the social.[99]

The physical dimension is at the root of the total pain experience; the person hurts, and the hurt is not going away. As time goes on, the pain begins to take on new dimensions. It may increase or decrease, but the uncertainty involved makes even a period of relief a time of tension in the expectation that pain will return. Bonica has shown that persistent pain produces a progressive physical deterioration because of lack of sleep and appetite as well as the frequent instance of excessive medication.[100] Likewise, one's pain threshold and tolerance are lowered as pain persists, thus heightening the experience of pain, which, in turn, continues to exert a negative influence. Understood in this way, it can correctly be said that pain itself contributes to, and is not merely a consequence of, dying.

The psychological dimension of pain is illustrated in the patient's suffering. Suffering is known to be physiologically distinct from the physical experience of pain.[101] The distinction can be seen here in the anguish that is brought on because of the pain. If the pain is poorly managed, the patient will become increasingly anxious and depressed,[102] even if the intensity of the pain does not increase. Similarly, when the pain persists, as it does in chronic pain, it is no longer seen as serving any useful purpose. Instead, the pain reinforces the lack of control experienced by the patient and the family. This may account for the incidence of hypochondriasis and a tendency to deny life problems unrelated to one's own physical behavior among people who suffer from chronic pain. These people also tend to have increased levels of neuroticism.[103]

The social effects of pain are equally as devastating. As the patient become more anxious, he/she may begin to act out that anxiety and frustration in anger, leading to the possibility or the perception of abandonment. As the patient becomes more depressed, he/she may begin to withdraw, adding to the sense of isolation. People experiencing pain often are unable to work, a reality that adds an economic stress to the situation, along with a feeling of dependency and uselessness. The physical appearance and behavior brought on by the person's pain and suffering also place an emotional stress on the family. This is perceived by the person and can further aggravate the ordeal.

A picture of this three-dimensional pain is found in Fig. 4.4[104] on the following page.

It should be noted that the physiological, psychological, and social impact of cancer pain on the person is greater than that of nonmalignant chronic pain. This results in a higher incidence of depression among cancer patients with pain.[105] This may also be true of persons who experience pain associated with AIDS. This depression, coupled with intractable pain, represents a state of helplessness on the part of the person, as well as an inability to cope with the disease, damage to the body, and the threat to life.

Bonica suggests that personality factors, distorted by pain, can be restored when that pain is controlled.[106] One way to facilitate this restoration, beyond the use of analgesics, is the practice of what Benoliel et al. call "staying."[107] Staying has to do with physical presence in care, being available for the patient in spite of the care giver's feelings of helplessness. To stay with the patient requires a deep conviction of the worth of what one is doing. This conviction becomes evident to the patient, who begins to grow in confidence that perhaps the pain can be controlled. The patient knows that attempts to control pain will not always be 100 percent successful. What the person needs is the confidence that complaints of pain will be heard, taken seriously, and attended to by another.

Pattern of Responses that Operates to Protect the Organism from Harm.
Pain is meant to initiate a series of responses with the purpose of protecting a person from harm. Because these responses are for the protection of the person as a whole, it is correct to say that they will be on the part of the person as a whole. The person as a whole, as all those characteristics discussed earlier, responds to the pain. This means that just as pain affects the physical, psychological, and social dimensions of the person, so will the body, psyche, and relationships of the person come to play a role in efforts to control pain.

Attempts to relieve a person from pain need to be directed toward the support of the person's own efforts to deal with the pain. Supportive counseling, tranquilizers, and/or antidepressants can frequently be used as effective complements to analgesics. It is important to take into consideration what the person thinks about his/her own pain, the underlying physical cause, the meaning to the individual, the context of the situation in which the pain is experienced, and the past experiences the person has had with pain, as well as the learning that accompanied these experiences. The goal will be to move away from a therapy that says, "I am going to take care of your pain," to "I am going to help you deal with your pain." This is

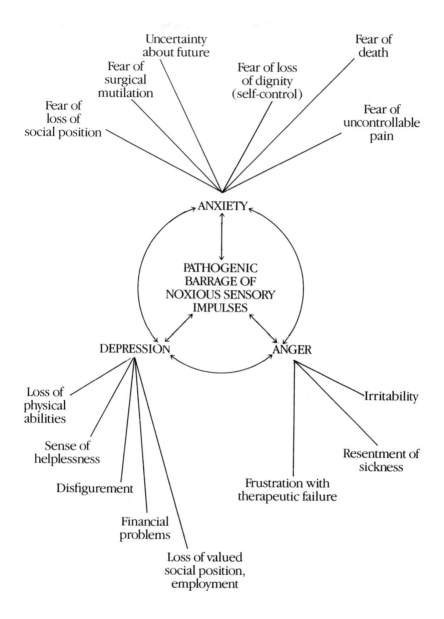

Fig. 4.4 Three Dimensions of Pain

Adapted from John J. Bonica, "Cancer Pain," in *The R.V.H. Manual on Palliative/Hospice Care,* eds. Ina Ajemian and Balfour M. Mount, Ayer Company Publishers, Salem, NII, 1982, p. 117.

accomplished by teaching new coping strategies or extending past ones. Pain will be relieved not merely by the administration of drugs. Pain is best relieved by assisting the person in coming to terms with his/her own pain.

Assessment of Pain

It should be obvious that a careful and accurate assessment of the person's pain is absolutely necessary if pain is to be controlled. An overall assessment will include the person's medical, psychological, financial, familial, social, cultural, religious, and philosophical status. The concern in this book will be primarily with the objective, physical reality of pain and its assessment. Although an overall assessment is needed, the immediate need to control the physical dimension of pain must be dealt with before some of the other psychosocial interventions will be possible.

In a physical assessment, the objective is to try to understand what the patient is experiencing and to examine the sites of pain in order to determine if pain is localized, diffuse, or referred. It is also important to determine if a particular activity alleviates or aggravates the pain, how sleep is affected, and whether or not the patient is taking any other medication that may affect the metabolism or medication used for pain.[108]

In this objective assessment, it is essential that the patient be allowed to offer his/her own ideas of what is happening. This gives a subjective assessment. One method of accomplishing this is to ask the person to complete a subjective and quantitative assessment of his/her pain. The *McGill-Melzack Pain Questionnaire* was developed for just this purpose.

This questionnaire lists three dimensions of pain: the sensory, affective, and evaluative. The patient uses these dimensions to specify the subjective pain experience. The questionnaire also includes an intensity scale, designed to provide a quantitative measure of clinical pain that can be treated statistically. The two measures derived from the questionnaire are the subjective *pain rating index (PRI)*, based on numerical values that are assigned to each word description, and the quantitative *present pain intensity (PPI)*, which is based on a scale of 0 through 5. The questionnaire also includes a front and back body diagram to allow the patient to indicate precisely where the pain is located.

It is also helpful for the staff to make their own assessment of the patient's pain. For this purpose, the PCU at Western Massachusetts Hospital in Westfield has established definitions of pain based on observable behavior:

Mild pain

• Patient appears relatively comfortable.

- Patient can move about or be moved without any facial grimacing or splinting of body parts.
- Patient sleeps well at night; needs to be awakened for medication and returns to sleep within 15 to 20 minutes.
- Appetite is good relative to state of disease.
- Patient appears to be reasonably outgoing.
- Few requests for increase or changes in pain medication.

Moderate pain

- Patient appears comfortable at times but also has periods of discomfort.
- Patient displays facial grimacing or splinting of body parts when moved; may stiffen in anticipation of being moved; grinds teeth together.
- Patient sleeps in naps but does not appear to sleep for long periods; is awake when medication is given at night and does not return to sleep easily; is restless.
- Appetite is poor relative to state of disease.
- Patient has periods of excessive irritability; displays decreased socialization.
- Infrequent requests for pain medication beyond prescribed regime.

Severe pain

- Patient appears restless most of the time.
- Patient displays facial grimacing, splinting, or stiffening of body parts; is unwilling or resistant to participate in even minimal movement; moans and grinds teeth.
- Patient sleeps poorly if at all; appears restless when asleep, moaning frequently.
- Appetite very poor or anorexic.
- Patient is unable or unwilling to carry on even minimal social interaction; displays extreme anxiety.
- Frequent requests for increase in or extra pain medication.

After the nurses' assessment is recorded, it is charted along with the patient's own assessment of pain. In this way, the unit has a consistent record of how adequately the patient's pain appears to be controlled, both from an objective and a subjective perspective.

On admission to the unit, an immediate assessment is made of the patient's pain. It is estimated that 75 percent of the patients at the PCU have pain that is not controlled at the time of admission. This may be the result of previous poor management of pain, the ambulance ride, the trauma of moving, or a combination of these factors. Efforts are made to bring this pain under control by analgesic dosages determined by titration. Titration refers to the process of determining the precise dose and frequency of an analgesic required to keep the plasma concentration of the analgesic at a level that will maintain relief, yet below levels of toxicity or sedation. This is always determined on an individual basis. Analgesics are never administered according to a purely statistical formulation of what should be given and when.

The method of titration used at the PCU is to prescribe dose ranges and administer the medication as dictated by the circumstances. For example, a dose range of 30 to 80 mg of Roxanol, a form of morphine, may be prescribed every four hours. This time frame is based on the duration of the clinical effect of the narcotic. Supplemental doses may be administered sometime within that time frame if required to keep the patient comfortable for the full amount of hours. The following regularly administered doses will be determined by how well the patient's pain was controlled by the previous dosage. If supplemental doses were needed for four hours of comfort, the regular dose will be increased. If the person experienced hallucinations or excessive sleepiness, it will be decreased. Periods of drowsiness or extended sleeping after the initial medication are, however, usually indicative of the patient's catching up on sleep due to the fatigue caused by the previously uncontrolled pain, not an overdose. The goal is to achieve the longest period of relief with the smallest dosage possible. It is estimated that a patient's pain can be controlled using this method of titration within 48 to 72 hours after admission. Once the pain is controlled, the analgesic is regularly administered at the determined dose to prevent the reemergence of pain.

Reassessment of the person's pain is made within hours if the pain is severe or within a day or two if moderate. This will help to determine if the medication is working consistently with any possible changes in the disease process and to ensure that side effects are kept to a minimum. Reassessment is also necessary because often relief of the primary pain allows a second and less severe pain to become apparent. When this happens, this secondary pain must also be addressed. For example, Twycross mentions an 85-year-old man with cancer of the prostate and pain in the right femur caused by a metastatic tumor. He was given aspirin and a narcotic analgesic for the pain. The next day he still complained of pain, although it was less severe. In questioning, it was learned that the site of the pain was the lower end of the abdomen. In fact, there was no femur pain at all. The dose of the narcotic was left unchanged, and an antacid was prescribed. The man enjoyed complete pain relief.[109]

Even after the initial management of a person's pain, the reassessment of symptoms continues throughout the person's stay. Depending on the influence that psychological factors have on the person's pain and any changes made in the environment, a person's need for medication may increase or decrease over time.

As death approaches, poor circulation and a slower metabolism sometimes result in drug accumulation, requiring a decrease in medication. External events, such as the noisy installation of new fire doors in the PCU in 1985, may result in an increase in the intensity of the pain experienced, requiring an increase in medication.

Use of Narcotics for Pain Management

The palliative therapies of surgery, radiation, and chemotherapy are often not effective or are contraindicated by the particular circumstances of a patient. In such cases, nonnarcotic analgesics are often used to bring the person's pain under control. These analgesics, however, are frequently ineffective for people with severe chronic pain. In these instances, a great deal of success has been obtained through the use of narcotic analgesics.

The use of narcotics in the United States is controversial, both morally and legally. Most of the controversy appears to be rooted in fears of adverse side effects such as dependence, tolerance, and addiction.[110] Most of these fears are founded on evidence gained from studies with animals, patients with acute pain who have been given single parenteral doses, and persons who have abused the drugs.[111] The application of this information to patients with chronic pain and to oral usage is questionable at best. As will be shown, physical dependence is not a problem in patients who are terminally ill; tolerance does not pose a clinical difficulty; and psychological addiction, except in cases when the person was previously addicted, is rare.

Dependence. The World Health Organization (WHO) has defined dependence as:

> *A state of psychic and sometimes also physical need, resulting from the interaction between a living organism and a drug, characterized by behavioral and other responses that always include a compulsion to take the drug on a continuous periodic basis in*

129

order to experience its psychic effects, and sometimes avoid the discomfort of its absence.[112]

Dependence has both a physical and a psychological dimension. For the sake of clarity, dependence will refer here only to the physical dimension of this need, leaving the psychological needs to be treated as the phenomenon of addiction.

Although the long-term use of narcotics with cancer patients remains a relatively unstudied area, evidence does suggest that physical dependence develops in the majority of patients within four weeks when the narcotic is given parenterally and less rapidly, and possibly to a lesser degree when given orally.[113] There is general medical agreement, however, that this physical dependence is not a practical problem for the person with terminal cancer who may require pain relief until death. Experience has also shown that the narcotic dose can be gradually reduced or even eliminated if it is no longer clinically required.[114] When the narcotic is reduced gradually, the person does not experience symptoms of withdrawal. According to Mount:

> *It is possible but not certain that physical dependence regularly occurs when oral morphine is used. ... If it occurs it does not prevent the downward adjustment of narcotic dose and even cessation of therapy when that is clinically feasible. Indeed, withdrawal reactions do not occur if the dose is tapered in stopping the narcotic even after periods of regular administration extending to years.*[115]

Tolerance. Tolerance refers to the state in which a person's body adjusts or becomes desensitized to the presence of the narcotic, thus requiring ever-increasing doses to achieve the same effect. Tolerance occurs with all narcotics. The risk involved is that the person will experience respiratory depression as a result of the larger doses required. This does not, however, appear to be a problem in the care of the terminally ill person.[116]

Although tolerance does pose a problem in cases of acute pain or when pain is of a psychological nature, it is less of a problem in people with severe chronic pain when appropriate doses are given. This is because people with chronic pain react differently to narcotics than do those who seek the euphoric effects of the drug or who receive it for pain of primarily psychogenic origin. It is believed that, in people with severe pain, the physiological processes differ from persons not experiencing this pain. This difference in the physiological state may result in a different pharmacological response. The clinical reality is that little tolerance develops in people in whom there is an active pain-producing process.[117]

Mount reports that, when administered properly, the narcotic morphine does not carry any of the dangers of tolerance. For example, the dose needed to induce respiratory depression is always higher than the dose necessary to control pain, so the impact of tolerance on the dosage, if it does occur, is negligible. In addition, the occurrence of tolerance peaks in most cases and usually ceases to be a factor after a few weeks.[118] Any increase in the dose that is required is attributable to a change in pathophysiology, such as the development of some new metastases or the collapse of a vertebra, not tolerance.[119]

Addiction. Addiction is the psychological dependence one may develop with the use of narcotics. Twycross defines it as "a compulsive or overpowering drive to take the drug in order to experience its psychological effects."[120] Addiction is not a problem in pain management for the terminally ill person who was not previously addicted.

At times, the phenomenon of addiction may appear to exist. This is sometimes seen in people who experience chronic pain but who are being treated as if they suffered from acute pain. That is, efforts are being made to relieve pain rather than prevent it. A routine of injections of inadequate amounts of narcotics given every four hours usually results in clock watching by the patient as fears begin to mount that the pain will return and become unbearable before the next injection. In such cases, true addiction does not exist. The patient, although demanding the drug, is not doing so out of a need or desire for psychological enjoyment but to obtain an hour or two of relief.

When used for their euphoric effects, narcotics do exert an addictive force on an individual. However, when narcotics are given regularly in adequate amounts so that pain and the fear of its recurrence are not in the forefront of the person's mind, the possibility that each drug-taking act will be reinforced is minimized.[121] The practice of undertreating is, in fact, more likely to encourage craving and psychological dependence than the regular administration of adequate doses.[122]

Adverse Reactions and Adjunct Medication. Narcotics are not without their side effects, and these also need to be controlled if pain is to be adequately relieved. Some patients will occasionally exhibit allergic reactions such as a rash or severe itching at the site of an injection of morphine. These are caused by a histamine release, and an antihistamine can be administered or the narcotic changed to one of a different structure. More common is the experience of constipation, nausea, and vomiting. This can be prevented with proper care and/or adjunct medication.

Drowsiness and somnolence are frequent side effects associated with the use of narcotics. This is especially true in palliative care when their use is first initiated. This can be partially explained by the fact that, when a person's pain has not been properly controlled, he/she will be exhausted from anxiety and lack of sleep. When the pain is brought under control by the proper use of narcotics, the person takes advantage of the relief and sleeps. In this case, the sleepiness is not caused by the narcotic, but by fatigue. With proper titration, a patient can remain alert and conscious even with narcotic analgesics. The dose required for pain relief is below that of sedation. Toxicity resulting from the accumulation of the narcotic in the body is not a practical problem in view of the brief half-life of drugs such as morphine,[123] the most frequently used narcotic for palliative pain control in the United States.

Somnolence is sometimes a part of the dying event itself. This may be caused by a withdrawal on the part of the person as he/she prepares to die. It may also result from the inability of the person to metabolize the narcotic properly. Patients who are actively dying often require less medication, and care needs to be taken that a dose larger than necessary is not given.

When somnolence occurs in the presence of persisting pain, the possibility that the pain is rooted in psychological factors, rather than in some physical cause, should be explored. In such cases, the somnolence may be the result of an overdose relative to the physical component of the pain. A lowering of the narcotic dose, an investigation of the nonphysical factors of the patient's pain, and the control of other symptoms are required.

Depression is an additional factor involved with the use of narcotics, although it is not certain if it is brought on by the protracted illness itself or is a side effect of long and continuous treatment with narcotics. When the person's depression is rooted in deep psychological factors or is medically induced, antidepressants could be considered.

A fear that is often expressed is respiratory depression. If the narcotic depressed the patient's respiratory function, death could be hastened. It is, however, extremely rare that such depression is of clinical significance when the narcotics are administered orally and in individually determined doses.[124] As with sedation, the dose required for palliation is below that necessary for respiratory depression, except for those patients with respiratory difficulties. In these cases, careful titration with attention to respiratory ventilation at each dose administered reduces the risks involved. In cases of need, a respiratory stimulant, such as amiphenazole, could be given.[125] Concerning the limited use of a stimulant, Mount reports that:

> *In treating several hundred patients over the past five and one half years, we have administered narcotic antagonists on only three*

*occasions when morphine was used as described: In one case
following an error in the dose of narcotic given by a nurse; in the
second case, probably unnecessarily, to a somnolent terminally ill
cancer patient who had longstanding chronic respiratory insuffi-
ciency; and in the third instance following respiratory arrest that
occurred as part of an idiosyncratic response to a low dose of
morphine.*[126]

A wide variety of narcotics are available including morphine, heroin
(known clinically as diamorphine), cocaine, methadone, meperidine,
anileridine, and levorphanol.[127] Although the most common narcotics used
today are morphine, diamorphine, and methadone, experience suggests
that, when regularly administered, oral morphine is the best choice in the
care of the terminally ill patient who experiences severe chronic pain,
particularly in cases of pain related to cancer.

The practice of using multiple drugs to treat cases of extreme pain
began late in the nineteenth century. Usually a mixture of morphine and
codeine was used.[128] Later mixtures substituted heroin for morphine. In
time, these mixtures took on nonmedical, social names such as "Mist
Euphoria," "Hospice Mix," "Saunders' Solution," "Euphoriant Solution," and
the "Brompton's Cocktail." Today, these practices are no longer considered
justified. Codeine, which may have been added as a local analgesic for the
throat as well as to relieve some of the side effects of morphine, is no longer
used because of its association with confusion and hallucinations. The
mixing of narcotics is considered by many to be irrational, since it offers no
pharmaceutic or therapeutic advantage.[129] The social naming of medication
has also been discouraged. The use of such names, although considered
"homey" by some, merely obscures the content of the analgesic.[130]

The use of heroin, which is currently illegal in the United States, is
often a subject of debate in matters of pain control. The question is raised as
to whether heroin is a more effective narcotic than morphine in pain
management. Like morphine, heroin has a duration of action of approximately four hours. It differs in potency, however, being just less than twice
that of morphine. Studies cited by Twycross suggest that this greater potency
ratio may be misleading.[131] Laboratory tests of the urinary excretions of
patients regularly receiving morphine and heroin show that heroin is
completely absorbed by the gastrointestinal tract, whereas morphine is only
two-thirds absorbed. This suggests that the apparent potency ratio of the
two drugs, administered orally, is in part only a reflection of the alimentary
absorption ratio of the two and not really a true reflection of potency
differences. It has also been noted that heroin quickly breaks down in vivo
to an intermediate stage before later breaking down to morphine. This

suggests that heroin itself has only a transient pharmacological action of its own. This adds support to the conclusion of many that, administered orally, morphine is as effective in pain management as heroin.[132]

Methadone may offer an alternative in management because it is highly soluble. This makes it possible to administer large doses of the narcotic parenterally in a small fluid volume. It can be given orally or parenterally with few side effects other than the nausea and constipation that usually accompany the use of any narcotic. Methadone has a duration of action of more than seven hours, allowing for longer periods between medication.

A disadvantage with methadone is the occurrence of accumulation, which raises the danger of toxicity and makes titration difficult. In view of this difficulty, Twycross reports that most physicians eventually switch the prescription of their patients receiving methadone to morphine or heroin.[133] There can also be a psychological advantage to switching from methadone to morphine. Some patients, once they learn to trust the new narcotic to control pain, prefer to receive medication more frequently than the every seven hours made possible by the methadone. The shorter interval between medication sometimes adds to a sense of security in pain control.

It can be concluded that, when other palliative therapies and nonnarcotic analgesics are not effective or feasible, the use of narcotic analgesics is appropriate for the control of chronic pain, even if the person is expected to live for an extended time. Morphine is the most common and useful of the narcotics available for most instances of severe chronic pain management with the terminally ill.

Three principles might be derived from this section on the use of narcotics:

1. Optimal doses should be determined by titration with respect to the individual, not by statistical analysis. Although large doses may be required, it should be remembered that doses for the control of acute pain are often insufficient in cases of chronic pain and that respiration, pulse rate, and other vital signs generally remain normal or are only slightly depressed.
2. It is generally better to begin with a high dose, with the intent to titrate downward. Unless the pain is brought under immediate control, efforts will be frustrated by the patient's increasing anxiety. The person's total pain must be addressed, and this can only be accomplished if the fear of pain is addressed.
3. Narcotics should be administered on a regularly scheduled basis. Narcotics are effective in the management of chronic pain because of their ability to block pain before it surfaces. Prevention of the

recurrence of pain lessens anxiety. In addition, it usually requires smaller doses of an analgesic to block pain than to relieve it once it is allowed to surface.

Although the use of narcotics has sometimes been referred to as bad management because it gives the patient a series of ups and downs and leads to addiction, clinical experience indicates that, with attention to detail, none of these need happen. With moderate to severe chronic pain, only narcotics provide adequate relief. They do so safely and with great benefit to the total relief of the person.

NUTRITION AND THE TERMINALLY ILL

The issue of maintaining adequate levels of nutritional and fluid support in people who are severely handicapped, terminally ill, irreversibly comatose, or in a persistent vegetative state is a difficult one. More than with other fatal illnesses or health crisis situations, cancer and AIDS place the question of feeding within the larger context of balancing the aggressive treatment of the disease with an acceptable quality of life. This is because with these diseases, the person is generally aware and conscious as the time of death approaches, and the therapies to treat the disease generally affect the person's nutritional levels as well as the desire or ability to eat. The question of discovering this balance introduces a measure of ambiguity in what is often seen as a nonquestion: one simply always feeds a patient. The current debate within the medical profession over the benefits of aggressive, nutritional support and the subjective aspects of anorexia and weight loss, which often afflict cancer and AIDS patients, adds to this ambiguity. One consequence of this is the heightened role that emotional factors now play in determining the meaning and use of artificial feeding for the patient, the family, and the medical profession.

There are many factors that raise the issue of the appropriateness of nutritional support for the dying person. These include the incidence of anorexia, nausea, vomiting, pain, changes in the sense of taste, reduced physical and emotional endurance, stomatitis, an altered metabolism, malabsorption and ascites, and difficulties with chewing and swallowing. For the person for whom cure is a reasonable hope, therapies that will bring about this cure demand good nutritional support. For the person who is not going to be cured, however, or who has suffered from these conditions for an extended time, there may no longer be any desire or ability to maintain adequate levels of nutrition. It is in this instance that the question emerges of whether or not nutritional support improves one's quality of life. It is at this point that well-being becomes the focus.

There are two principal medical procedures that provide artificial nutritional support. The first delivers liquids through a tube into a functioning gastrointestinal tract. This can be done in two ways. One method is to insert a nasogastric tube through the nose and esophagus into the stomach. At other times a second method is used, in which a gastrotomy tube is inserted through a surgical incision in the abdominal wall directly into the stomach. A nasogastric tube is inexpensive, but it may lead to pneumonia. Further, it is often annoying to the patient and family, sometimes requiring that the patient be restrained to prevent its removal. A gastrotomy is generally a simple procedure. Once the incision is healed, it requires simple care, is less visible and therefore esthetically more acceptable, and presents no danger of pneumonia.

The second procedure to maintain levels of nutrition and fluids is by intravenous (IV) feeding and hydration. This can be done most simply through a peripheral IV line that delivers fluids directly into the blood. An IV setup is useful only for temporary efforts to improve hydration and electrolyte concentrations. It is not useful in providing a balanced diet. A more complicated but nutritionally more effective procedure is the insertion of a catheter into one of the main veins of the chest. This procedure entails a greater risk and is prone to infection. Both methods require hospitalization and often also necessitate restraining the patient.

Feeding, as a natural human act, involves the placing of food into the mouth, the chewing of it, the food being swallowed through the esophagus, and the food passing into the stomach and intestines, where it is digested. Medical intervention circumvents this natural procedure dramatically. This results in very different meanings being assigned to the eating process, raising the issue of psychological factors.

Peteet et al. found in a study conducted at the Sidney Farber Cancer Institute, Boston, that a patient's willingness to accept artificial feeding was influenced by emotional factors that appeared to be related to the illness and to personality factors.[134] With respect to the illness itself, it was shown that for many patients, the loss of appetite, weight, and body image were the primary threats that cancer posed to the person's sense of self and autonomy. The wasting away of the body brought on by the disease became closely associated with, if not seen as identical to, the sickness. That is, the wasting away of the body was seen as *being* the illness rather than a *result* of the illness. Artificial nutrition, therefore, became viewed as a way of combatting the disease, and its acceptability was often accompanied by an unusually high expectation for cure. From the family's perspective, feeding was generally equated with caring. The patient's acceptance or refusal of this care had implications for the whole family, not just the patient.

With respect to personality factors, three patterns were especially common. With the demoralized or depressed person, the loss of confidence in the ability to eat was part of a more profound loss of confidence in him/herself. Efforts to feed the person that did not first address these fears often resulted in increasing the person's dependency, fear of helplessness, and anxiety. Patients with strong independent personalities, on the other hand, sometimes made an issue of eating and artificial feeding in order to maintain a sense of control. Pressure from the family or the medical staff could provoke a crisis. Finally, extreme or rigid attitudes toward artificial eating and weight loss sometimes reflected an unusual anxiety or feelings of helplessness over a worsening prognosis. At issue here was not so much the question of eating but of psychological preparation for death.

Appropriate care makes it necessary to discover and pursue the balance between adequate nutritional support and well-being. It is necessary to discover the meaning of eating and artificial feeding for the person and the family. This entails an assessment of the person's personality, the family's ways of relating, and the effects of stress on the emotional state of everyone involved. Obvious emotional conflicts should be addressed directly to minimize their influence on nutritional decisions.

Of great importance is care based specifically on the patient's needs, which often vary greatly from the needs of the others involved. If the person needs to be in control, then this control must be given so that the feeding does not become symbolic of a greater issue. Any patient whose refusal to eat is indicative of depression and demoralization needs encouragement and support. It should not be forgotten, however, that the person who is dying often has an interest in dying. Because feeding is life sustaining, its relative unimportance to the person is valid, even if difficult for care givers to accept.

It is clear that the question of feeding the terminally ill person is not without its ambiguities. Artificial feeding may be the issue in question or it may be the manifestation of other issues that need to be addressed. In any case, merely inserting a nasogastric tube or initiating an IV line as a standard course of treatment for the terminally ill person is not appropriate. The psychological meaning of artificial feeding for patients and their families has direct implications for improving both their cooperation and their well-being. If these issues are not addressed, suffering will continue even if adequate levels of nourishment are maintained.

Simply to discover the meaning of feeding in a particular instance does not solve the issue. It might still be questioned whether the medical reality indicates, regardless of the psychological meaning attached to it, that maintaining adequate levels of nutrition and hydration are necessary in a particular instance. It may be that this does not offer the patient a real improvement over what would otherwise be faced. Lynn and Childress suggest three situations in which artificial means of maintaining adequate levels of foods and fluids might be appropriately withheld or withdrawn[135]:

1. *Futile or dangerous treatment.* For example, a patient with severe congestive heart failure develops cancer of the stomach and a fistula that delivers food from the stomach to the colon without its being passed through the intestines and being absorbed. Feeding is technically possible, but little will be absorbed. An IV line cannot be tolerated because the fluids would be too much for the heart. The patient is going to die with or without treatment, and efforts to sustain life may even increase discomfort. The medical fact that the protein balance is negative or the blood serum is concentrated should not cause one to lose sight of the fact that, medically, efforts to sustain life will be futile or even dangerous.

2. *No possibility of benefit.* Some patients will be diagnosed as being permanently without consciousness, as in the case of anencephaly, persistent vegetative states, and some preterminal comas. It is difficult to determine that any medical intervention is going to be of either benefit or harm to the person. Although palliation of symptoms is always mandated, efforts to sustain life may be in the interest of the family or the healthcare team rather than in the interest of the patient.

3. *Disproportionate burden.* The most difficult cases are those in which normal nutritional states can be restored in the patient, but only with severe burden. In such cases, the treatment may be futile in the long term. To improve nutrition and hydration is not always to the benefit of the patient. Treatments that restore a person's body to optimal nutritional levels are never without some side effects, and their benefits always fall short of the ideal. Further, many patients who are most likely to be malnourished or dehydrated are also more likely to suffer the most serious side effects of the nutritional therapies previously mentioned.

Patients who are allowed to die without artificial nutrition and hydration may die more comfortably than those who receive conventional amounts of IV hydration.[136] Instances of terminal pulmonary edema, nausea, and mental confusion are more likely when patients have been treated to maintain fluids and nutrition right up to the time of death. Thus, those patients whose need for nutritional support arises only near the time of death may be harmed. It is not at all clear that these patients gain any benefit from a slightly prolonged life with a lessened quality.

This reflection also applies to persons whose life could be lengthened considerably by the medical intervention of nutritional support. This includes patients with fairly severe dementia, for whom the required restraints would be a constant source of anxiety, irritation, and struggle. Any sedation that would be required to tolerate the feeding would certainly make whatever time is gained of little value. Whether a longer life with constraints or a shorter life with a freedom of spirit, if not movement, is preferable is a question that needs to be addressed in these issues.

The goal of palliative care is to give as much nutritional support as desired and tolerated by the person in an attractive and social setting. This is an aspect of comfort and care for the patient. After that, the question of nutrition is an open one. At times, a nasogastric tube will be removed because the patient no longer chooses to gain more nutrition than he/she can take orally. At other times, a cup of tea will be given to relieve symptoms of dryness and thirst because it tastes good, even though it will not adequately address dehydration. Other patients might request and be given popcorn to eat, knowing full well that it may cause them some discomfort the next day.

In questions of nutrition, palliative care seeks always to achieve the highest quality of life available to the person. When this can best be done by artificial feeding, then it is the appropriate course. When the quality of life of the person is better served by refraining from these medical interventions, then this is viewed as an acceptable course of action to be chosen by the person or, in cases of incompetence, by those legally and morally responsible. Although it may never serve the interests of the person to become malnourished, it may serve his/her interests in quality of life and well-being to not receive treatment to alleviate the malnutrition.

NOTES

1. Alexander S.D. Spiers, "The Palliative Management of Cancer Patients," in *Cancer: A Manual for Practitioners,* 5th ed., ed. Blake Cady, American Cancer Society, Boston, 1978, p. 307 (hence referred to as *Cancer: A Manual*).
2. Balfour M. Mount, "Keynote: Introduction to Death and Dying Services in the Acute Care Hospital," delivered at the Fourth International Seminar on Terminal Care, Montreal, Canada, 1983. A tape of Mount's address was made available to the author through the courtesy of Jo-Anne Wallace, Director of St. Joseph's Hospice, Nashua, NH.
3. Melvyn P. Richter, "Palliative Radiation Therapy," *Clinical Care of the Terminal Cancer Patient,* eds. Barrie R. Cassileth and Peter A. Cassileth, Lea & Febiger, Philadelphia, 1982, p. 65 (hence referred to as *Clinical Care*).
4. Spiers, p. 307.

5. Ina Ajemian, "General Principles of Symptomatic Management," in *The R.V.H. Manual on Palliative/Hospice Care,* eds. Ina Ajemian and Balfour M. Mount, Ayer Company Publishers, Salem, NH, 1982, p. 184 (hence referred to as *R.V.H. Manual*).

6. Ajemian, p. 184.

7. Mount.

8. Cicely M. Saunders, "Appropriate Treatment, Appropriate Death," in *The Management of Terminal Disease,* ed. Cicely M. Saunders, Edward Arnold Publishers Ltd., London, 1978, p. 1 (hence referred to as *Management*).

9. See Richter, p. 66; Spiers, pp. 307-308; and Thelma D. Bates, "Radiotherapy in Terminal Care," in *Management,* p. 124.

10. J. Englebert Dunphy, "Annual Discourse: On Caring for the Patient with Cancer," in *Cancer: A Manual,* p. 339.

11. K.C. Calman, "Physical Aspects," in *Management,* p. 38.

12. Calman, pp. 38-39.

13. Dunphy, p. 344.

14. Elisabeth Kübler-Ross, *On Death and Dying,* MacMillan, New York, 1969, p. 30. See also Elisabeth Kübler-Ross, *Questions and Answers on Death and Dying,* MacMillan, New York, 1974, pp. 12 and 28.

15. Joan Craven and Florence S. Wald, "Hospice Care for Dying Patients," *American Journal of Nursing* 75, 1975, pp. 1816-1822, at 1819.

16. To ensure a patient's privacy, information is never given over the telephone concerning a patient's condition. Callers are always asked to identify themselves to give the patient the opportunity to screen calls if desired. Unwelcome visitors are told that the patient is unavailable.

17. One difficulty that physical therapy raises is the false hope of a cure because of its identification with rehabilitation. With respect to respiratory therapy, there are no ventilators in the PCU. Therapy consists primarily of the use of an oxygen updraft or bronchodialator, which dilates the bronchial passages to ease breathing. Aerosols are sometimes used for humidification, and chest percussion assists in removing phlegm.

18. Barbara M. Sourkes, *The Deepening Shade: Psychological Aspects of Life-Threatening Illness,* University of Pittsburgh Press, Pittsburgh, 1982, p. 79: "It is worth noting here that there is an essential difference between the use of conventional methods of anticancer therapy in patients with early disease, and in those with terminal disease. In the first circumstance, treatment is used to eradicate the tumor in the hope of cure; in the latter it is used for palliation."

19. Sourkes, p. 79; see also Calman, p. 38.

20. C. Murray Parkes, "Psychological Aspects," in *Management,* p. 46.

21. Calman, p. 37.

22. For a listing of potential problems, causes, emotional and social objectives, and possible therapies in symptom control, see Ajemian, pp. 187-198.

23. Other therapies, such as immunotherapy and hormone therapy, are not discussed here because of their more limited application. For studies indicating the continued development and possible future application of these, see Steven A. Rosenberg, et al., "Observations on the Systemic Administration

of Autologous Lymphokine-Activated Killer Cells and Recombinant Interleu-kin-2 to Patients with Metastatic Cancer," *The New England Journal of Medicine* 313, 1985, pp. 1485-1492; Sidney R. Cooperband, "Immunology: Overview and Future Prospects," in *Cancer: A Manual*, pp. 71-79; Peter J. Mozden and Blake Cady, "Overall Principles of Cancer Management. V. Hormone Therapy," in *Cancer: A Manual*, pp. 68-70; Harmon J. Eyre, "Advances in Cancer Management," *Proceedings of the National Conference on Practice, Education, and Research in Oncology Social Work—1984*, American Cancer Society, Boston, 1984, pp. 1-4 (hence referred to as *Proceedings of the National Conference*); and Edward Sylvester, *Target: Cancer*, Charles Scribner's Sons, New York, 1986.

24. Not all tumors are operable. The tumor's size, awkward or dangerous location, or the presence of tentacle-like extensions wrapped around other tissues may make removal clinically impossible. A tumor may also be described as inoperable if evidence of extensive growth or distant metastases make the prognosis so poor that any surgery, even though technically possible, is essentially futile. See Eyre, p. 1; the determination of tumor status as operable or inoperable relies to some extent on a physiological and psychological evaluation of the patient as well. In the former, for example, a pneumonectomy should generally not be performed on a patient who does not have adequate pulmonary reserve. In the latter, a mastectomy may be ruled out in the case of a woman with severely disturbed marital or sexual relationships. In both cases, alternative therapies exist. See also Omar T. Pace and Blake Cady, "Overall Principles of Cancer Management. II. Surgery," in *Cancer: A Manual*, pp. 43-48.

25. Pace and Cady, p. 45.

26. Eyre, p. 2.

27. Surgical treatment after a failure of radiation therapy is generally successful, whereas radiation following an unsuccessful attempt to remove the tumor surgically is generally unsuccessful. See Pace and Cady, p. 46; and Steven A. Rosenberg, "Combined-Modality Therapy of Cancer: What Is It and When Does It Work?" *The New England Journal of Medicine* 312, 1985, pp. 1512-1514.

28. Pace and Cady, p. 46.

29. Although pain is the symptom most often feared, it is not always the most difficult to control. Opinions vary, but nausea and vomiting are certainly among the most difficult.

30. Michael R. Williams, "The Place of Surgery in Terminal Care," in *Management*, p. 134.

31. Williams, p. 134.

32. Martin B. Levene, "Overall Principles of Cancer Management. III. Radiation Therapy," in *Cancer: A Manual*, pp. 49 and 56.

33. Levene, p. 56.

34. Poorly oxygenated cells within a tumor may result in a small cluster of viable cancer cells from which a recurrence may develop. See Levene, p. 51.

35. Levene, p. 52.

36. However, radiation therapy could be considered in the case of a collapsing cervical dorsal vertebra, even if this condition is not causing any pain, as a way

of preventing possible incontinence and paralysis. See Thelma D. Bates, "Radiotherapy in Terminal Care," in *Management,* p. 119; and Levene, p. 53.

37. Richter, p. 65.
38. Some tumors, such as most bone and soft tissue sarcomas, cerebral gliomas, and malignant melanomas, resist radiation and therefore are unlikely to respond to palliative doses. See Bates, p. 120.
39. Of the normal tissues, the gastrointestinal tract is one of the most sensitive to radiation. Large volumes of radiation to the abdomen will generally result in nausea and diarrhea, and small palliative doses of radiation to the region of the epigastrium or upper lumbar vertebrae will often result in nausea and vomiting. Most people believe that all radiation therapy is invariably associated with nausea and vomiting or diarrhea. This is not the case. Wide-field radiation of the chest, head, or limbs, for example, is generally only accompanied by a sense of fatigue during the first few hours after each treatment. See Bates, p. 120.
40. All tissues vary in response to radiation, but there is a limit to the total dosage any tissue can tolerate, even if that dosage is spread over many years. See Bates, p. 120.
41. Bates, p. 119.
42. There are two methods of palliative therapy. In the *short course,* individual doses of greater than 200 rads are given over less than two weeks. This course of therapy is appropriate when there is rapid tumor growth, when there is evidence of an early dissemination of the tumor following definitive treatment, or when the patient has a life expectancy of three months or less. In the *protracted course,* conventional doses of less than 200 rads are given over an extended period. This course of therapy is used when the patient has a life expectancy greater than three months, the tumor is associated with little or no pain, the tumor mass is greater than 10 × 10 cm, and there is a solitary metastasis associated with a controlled primary tumor. It is also used for locally extensive tumors of the head and neck as well as for those of the female genitourinary tract. See Richter, pp. 67-68.
43. Richter, p. 69.
44. Richter, p. 69.
45. In cases of metastases to the brain, the patient's ability to move about and the type of primary tumor may influence the ultimate prognosis. For example, patients who are ambulatory tend to live longer than those who are restricted, and patients with a primary breast tumor tend to live longer (21-week average) than those with a primary lung tumor (12-week average). See Richter, p. 70; see also Bruce B. Borgelt, "The Palliation of Brain Metastases: Final Results of the First Two Studies by the Radiation Therapy Oncology Group," *International Journal of Radiation Oncology, Biology & Physics* 6, 1980, pp. 1-9.
46. For a historical perspective of the development and use of chemotherapy, see John H. Glick, "Palliative Chemotherapy: Risk/Benefit Ratio," in *Clinical Care,* pp. 53-56.
47. Thelma D. Bates and Thérèse Vanier, "Palliation by Cytotoxic Chemotherapy and Hormone Therapy," in *Management,* p. 125.

48. Paul C. Hetzel, Marvin L. Hoovis, and Sheldon D. Kaufman, "Overall Principles of Cancer Management. IV. Chemotherapy," in *Cancer: A Manual,* pp. 59-60.
49. Hetzel et al., p. 59; Glick, pp. 55-57.
50. Glick, p. 55.
51. Hetzel et al., p. 61.
52. Hetzel et al., p. 61.
53. Hetzel et al., pp. 62 and 66.
54. Bates and Vanier, p. 125.
55. Bates and Vanier, p. 125.
56. Glick, pp. 53 and 57.
57. Bates and Vanier, p. 126.
58. "Candidate AIDS Vaccine," *Science* 235, 1987, p. 1575.
59. "Candidate AIDS Vaccine," p. 1575.
60. Kenneth H. Mayer and Steven M. Opal, "Therapeutic Approaches for AIDS and HIV Infection," *Rhode Island Medical Journal* 70, 1987, pp. 27-33.
61. Gene Robinson, Samuel E. Wilson, and Russell A. Williams, "Surgery in Patients with Acquired Immunodeficiency Syndrome," *Archives of Surgery* 122, 1987, pp. 170-175.
62. See C.M. Reichert, T.J. O'Leary, and D.L. Levens, "Autopsy Pathology in the Acquired Immune Deficiency Syndrome," *American Journal of Pathology* 112, 1983, pp. 375-382.
63. Williams, p. 134.
64. Robinson et al., p. 173.
65. Myron P. Nobler, Mary Ellen Leddy, and Sun H. Huh, "The Impact of Palliative Irradiation on the Management of Patients with Acquired Immune Deficiency Syndrome," *Journal of Clinical Oncology* 5, 1987, pp. 107-112.
66. Robinson et al., p. 173, citing J.W. Curran, W.M. Morgan, A.M. Hardy, et al., "The Epidemiology of AIDS: Current Status and Future Prospects," *Science* 229, 1985, pp. 1352-1357; see also Michael Marmor et al., "Kaposi's Sarcoma in Homosexual Men: A Seroepidemiologic Case-Control Study," *Annals of Internal Medicine* 100, 1984, pp. 809-815.
67. Jay S. Cooper, MD; Peter R. Fried, MD, "Defining the role of radiation therapy in the management of Epidemic Kaposi's Sarcoma," *International Journal of Radiation Oncology, Biology & Physics* 13(1), January, 1987, pp. 35-39.
68. Margaret A. Fischl et al., "The Efficacy of Azidothymidine (AZT) in the Treatment of Patients with AIDS and AIDS-Related Complex," *The New England Journal of Medicine* 317, 1987, pp. 185-191.
69. National Institute of Health (NIH) Conference, "Developmental Therapeutics and the Acquired Immunodeficiency Syndrome," *Annals of Internal Medicine* 106, 1987, pp. 568-581.
70. Douglas D. Richman et al., "The Toxicity of Azidothymidine (AZT) in the Treatment of Patients with AIDS and AIDS-Related Complex," *The New England Journal of Medicine* 317, 1987, pp. 192-197.
71. See also Harry Hollander, "Practical Management of Common AIDS-Related Medical Problems," *Western Journal of Medicine* 146, 1987, pp. 237-240.
72. Centers for Disease Control, "Update: Acquired Immunodeficiency Syn-

drome—United States," *Mortality and Morbidity Weekly Report* 35, 1986, p. 542.

73. NIH Conference, pp. 575-576.
74. NIH Conference, p. 576.
75. NIH Conference, p. 576.
76. Deborah M. Barnes, "Brain Damage by AIDS Under Active Study," *Science* 235, 1987, pp. 1574-1577; see also Joseph R. Berger, "Neurologic Complications of Human Immunodeficiency Virus Infection: What Diagnostic Features To Look For," *Postgraduate Medicine* 81, 1987, pp. 72-77.
77. Gregory L. Clark and Harry V. Vinters, "Dementia and Ataxia in a Patient with AIDS," *The Western Journal of Medicine* 146, 1987, pp. 68-72.
78. Carmelita U. Tuazon and Ann M. Labriola, "Management of Infections and Immunological Complications of Acquired Immunodeficiency Syndrome (AIDS): Current and Future Prospects," *Drugs* 33, 1987, p. 68.
79. Matthew Loscalzo, "Pain and Anxiety Control," *Proceedings of the National Conference,* p. 22.
80. Norman Cousins, *Anatomy of an Illness as Perceived by the Patient: Reflections on Healing and Regeneration,* Bantam Books, New York, 1979, p. 107.
81. Cousins, p. 107.
82. Robert G. Twycross, "Relief of Pain," in *Management,* p. 65; and Jeanne Q. Benoliel and Dorothy M. Crowley, *The Patient in Pain: New Concepts,* American Cancer Society, New York, 1974, p. 2.
83. See Twycross, "Relief of Pain," p. 66; Benoliel and Crowley, p. 3; and Anne Munley, *The Hospice Alternative: A New Context for Death and Dying,* Basic Books, New York, 1983, p. 20. It has been estimated that 20 percent of those patients who die of a tumor-related disease experience severe chronic pain; see Arthur G. Lipman, "Drug Therapy in Cancer Pain," *Cancer Nursing* 3, 1980, pp. 39-46.
84. Lipman, p. 39.
85. For a study showing the lack of pain control education in medical schools, the mismanagement of cancer pain, and the lack of knowledge concerning the basic mechanism and physiopathology of cancer pain, see John J. Bonica, "Cancer Pain," in *R.V.H. Manual,* pp. 118-128.
86. *Taber's Cyclopedic Medical Dictionary,* F.A. Davis, Philadelphia, 1985, p. 1206.
87. Benoliel and Crowley, p. 3.
88. See Patrick D. Wall, "On the Relation of Injury to Pain," *Pain* 6, 1979, pp. 253-264.
89. See John J. Bonica, "Importance of the Problem," in *Advances in Pain Research and Therapy,* vol. 2, eds. John J. Bonica et al., Raven Press, New York, 1979, pp. 1-12.
90. Ronald Melzack, "Current Concepts of Pain," in *R.V.H. Manual,* p. 96; and Loscalzo, p. 23. For example, religious guilt may play a role in the experience of pain. Although it is not possible to determine if guilt makes pain more intense, it does make it more difficult for the person to participate effectively in managing the pain when that pain is viewed as a form of punishment. In one case, a woman refused adequate medication, trusting that God would take care

of her. When her hopes were not realized, her disappointment made pain control nearly impossible.

91. Twycross, "Relief of Pain," p. 68.
92. Lipman, pp. 39-40; see also Loscalzo, p. 23.
93. Melzack, p. 96.
94. Loscalzo, p. 22.
95. Twycross, "Relief of Pain," p. 71.
96. Once pain is allowed to surface, the antagonistic reaction between the pain and the analgesic makes control more difficult, usually necessitating larger doses. Preventive care eliminates the fear of recurrence and the corresponding increase in pain intensity through anxiety and bodily tension. See Benoliel and Crowley, p. 18-19.
97. Twycross, "Relief of Pain," p. 72.
98. Lipman, p. 40.
99. Lipman, p. 40.
100. Bonica, "Cancer Pain," p. 115.
101. See David Bakan, *Disease, Pain, and Sacrifice: Toward A Psychology of Suffering,* Beacon Press, Chicago, 1971.
102. William M. Markel, and Virginia Sinon, "The Hospice Concept," *American Cancer Society Professional Education Publication,* American Cancer Society, Boston, 1978, p. 5; depression exists naturally in 20 to 25 percent of the total cancer population. See also Melzack, p. 97.
103. Bonica, "Cancer Pain," p. 115.
104. Bonica, "Cancer Pain," p. 117.
105. Bonica, "Cancer Pain," p. 117.
106. Bonica, "Cancer Pain," p. 117.
107. Benoliel and Crowley, p. 7.
108. Benoliel and Crowley, p. 6; and Markel et al., pp. 6-7.
109. Twycross, "Relief of Pain," p. 71.
110. Markel and Sinon, p. 5.
111. Joan Craven and Florence S. Wald, "Hospice Care for Dying Patients," *American Journal of Nursing* 75, 1975, p. 1818; Twycross, "Relief of Pain," pp. 82-83; and Balfour M. Mount, "Narcotic Analgesics in the Treatment of Pain of Advanced Malignant Disease," in *R.V.H. Manual,* pp. 148-149.
112. Mount, "Narcotic Analgesics," p. 156.
113. Mount, "Narcotic Analgesics," p. 156.
114. Craven and Wald, p. 1818; Lipman, p. 42; see also Robert G. Twycross, "Clinical Experience with Diamorphine in Advanced Malignant Disease," *International Journal of Clinical Pharmacology, Therapy and Toxicology* 7, 1974, pp. 197-198.
115. Mount, "Narcotic Analgesics," p. 156.
116. Munley, p. 21; see also Craven and Wald, p. 1818; Mount, "Narcotic Analgesics," p. 152; Cicely M. Saunders, "Patient Care: An Introduction," *Topics in Therapeutics,* ed. D.W. Vere, Pitman Press, London, 1978, pp. 72-110; and Balfour M. Mount, Ina Ajemian, and J.F. Scott, "Use of the Brompton Mixture in

Treating the Chronic Pain of Malignant Disease," *CMA Journal* 115, 1976, pp. 122-124.

117. Lipman, p. 42.
118. Mount, "Narcotic Analgesics," pp. 150, 155-156.
119. Mount, "Narcotic Analgesics," p. 150.
120. Twycross, "Relief of Pain," p. 82; see also Mount, "Narcotic Analgesics," p. 156.
121. Craven and Wald, p. 1818.
122. Munley, p. 21.
123. Mount, "Narcotic Analgesics," p. 156.
124. Twycross reports that "patients with tachypnea often feel better if, for example, the respiratory rate is reduced from 40 to 25 breaths a minute. With this observation in mind, one could consider raising the dose of diamorphine or morphine, even if pain is controlled, in order to ease dyspnea." Twycross, "Relief of Pain," p. 79; see also Mount, "Narcotic Analgesics," p. 154.
125. Twycross, "Relief of Pain," p. 79.
126. Mount, "Narcotic Analgesics," p. 154.
127. Lipman, p. 46. Experiments with marijuana have not been shown to be of significant benefit to most patients; see Sidney Cohen, "Marijuana, Does It Have a Possible Therapeutic Use?" *Journal of the American Medical Association* 240, 1978, pp. 1761-1763.
128. For a brief history of the use of multiple narcotic drugs, see Lipman, pp. 43-44.
129. Lipman, p. 43.
130. Twycross, "Relief of Pain," p. 75.
131. Twycross, "Relief of Pain," pp. 76-77.
132. Balfour M. Mount, "Correspondence: A letter to the editor of the *CMA Journal*," reprinted in *R.V.H. Manual,* pp. 165-166; Lipman, p. 46; William C. Farr, "Should Heroin Be Available for Pain?" *Journal of the American Medical Association* 241, 1979, pp. 882-883; and Mount, "Narcotic Analgesics," p. 150. Heroin does have a practical, although not pharmacological, advantage over morphine, found in the greater solubility of its hydrochloride. This allows smaller volume injections. See also Twycross, "Relief of Pain," p. 77.
133. Twycross, "Relief of Pain," p. 78.
134. John R. Peteet et al., "Psychological Aspects of Artificial Feeding in Cancer Patients," *Journal of Parenteral and Enteral Nutrition* 5, 1981, pp. 138-140.
135. Joanne Lynn and James F. Childress, "Must Patients Always Be Given Food and Water?" *The Hastings Center Report* 13, 1983, pp. 17-21.
136. Joyce V. Zerwekh, "The Dehydration Question," *Nursing '83* 13, 1983, pp. 47-51.

5 Morally Responsible Care for the Terminally Ill

This final chapter will put forward those ethical principles that are operative in the morally appropriate care of the terminally ill. Their foundation is based on the understanding of the person and the paradigm for well-being proposed earlier in this book and flow out of the medical reality as it has been presented. These principles reflect the needs of the person in health. Insights into how these needs are most appropriately addressed are drawn from the previous discussion concerning the different modalities of healthcare, as well as from the comparison of aggressive or curative therapy with palliative therapy as they are presently practiced.

In traditional healthcare ethics, the principle of totality, the distinction between ordinary and extraordinary, as well as the notions of proportionate and disproportionate means, have been helpful in defining appropriate medical care. The advancement of medical technology, however, has often obscured an understanding of the person as a patient and made it difficult to determine exactly what is meant by these expressions in particular situations. The principles derived from the paradigm of well-being and the practice of palliative care as described here seek to address this difficulty by distinguishing the total and sometimes hidden needs of the person from the presenting, more obvious needs. It is the total need of the person that gives insight into the discernment of appropriate medical interventions. It is my contention that the total need of the person is that of being brought beyond health or sickness to well-being. This alone allows the person to once again pursue the human task of placing or discovering meaning in life.

The ethical principles of healthcare suggested here will, for the most part, be articulated within the context of care for the terminally ill. Many of these principles are self-evident, flowing logically from what has been put forward in the preceding chapters. Others, such as those having to do with the value of life, the maintenance of adequate levels of hydration and

147

nutrition, and the use of narcotics for pain control, are more controversial. Although I believe that these principles are justified by this work as a whole, I will include here a somewhat broader discussion to demonstrate that the conclusions I have reached are grounded within contemporary ethical thought.

These principles will lead to a final statement on the ethical appropriateness of palliative care for the terminally ill. Morally responsible care will be that care that allows the person to move beyond suffering to well-being as he/she lives out and brings meaning to his/her dying. I would suggest, however, that these same principles apply equally in acute and chronic healthcare settings.

ETHICAL PRINCIPLES OF CARE FOR THE TERMINALLY ILL

The "person" is primary in all things.

The practice of medicine always involves persons. It is the person who becomes ill. Persons are all unique in who they are. Although it is possible to make a list of those characteristics that make up a person, it is never possible to make a complete or definitive list. Further, any list of characteristics must also allow for the aspect of integration. The person is not a collection of characteristics, but the bringing into a meaningful whole of those characteristics. As has been shown, individuals integrate who they are as persons differently.

I have chosen to speak of this integration to wholeness as a state of well-being. That is, a person enjoys well-being when he/she is able to integrate, to the extent possible, his/her life situation into him/herself. In other words, well-being has to do with being at one with the self as who the person is in the world in which he/she lives. If individuals integrate themselves as persons differently, well-being will be different for each person. Well-being can only be defined as an integrated wholeness of the person. It is not possible to describe exactly of what that will consist for people in general.

The antithesis of well-being I have called suffering. *Suffering* is that state in which the person perceives that his/her personal integrity is threatened by some outside force over which he/she has no control, a force that will ultimately destroy the person. Because the person is a uniquely integrated whole, all threats to that whole will be perceived in a unique way. Different people become ill differently even if they have the same disease. Further, people will suffer differently, even if the objective reality that induces that suffering, cancer or AIDS, for example, is the same. Because each person is integrated differently, threats to that integration will be perceived differently; thus the suffering will be different. The clinical approach taken to relieve that suffering must likewise be different.

There is nothing generic about health and sickness, wellness and suffering. Each is a uniquely personal experience. Decisions made to relieve suffering will always have to be made in the concrete reality of the person involved and not according to an abstract norm or general principle. Norms and principles offer insight and are useful. They cannot, however, be absolute.

Such an approach will necessarily involve some ambiguity. This cannot be avoided. Whenever we are dealing with persons, there will always be some ambiguity arising out of the particular uniqueness of the persons involved. In this context, that particular uniqueness lies in the way in which a person is integrated with him/herself in wholeness or well-being. Because persons are unique in their integration, they will also be unique in the way that integrity is threatened, and therefore in the way they suffer.

The moral imperative is to relieve suffering and to facilitate the living person in achieving well-being.

When a person presents him/herself as a patient, he/she does so as a person in need. As such, the patient places a moral demand on another. Once the need is expressed, there is a moral imperative to address that need. Such is clearly the teaching of the Judeo-Christian tradition, expressed in such readings as Genesis 4:8-16, which confirms that we are each other's keepers; the eschatological discourse of Matthew 25:31-46, indicating that our treatment of one another is our treatment of the Lord; and Luke 10:25-37, which teaches that all people are to become neighbors to each other.[1] When the presentation of need is made, there is an imperative to respond.

Traditionally it would be said that the person presents him/herself as a patient needing medical care to return to health. This is most effectively accomplished through the use of physical or psychological interventions aimed at relieving the problem that causes the ill health. This can, however, be too narrow a concept. Health has to do with the integration of the whole person. This is so much the case that I have suggested, for clarity, that the term *health* be used to apply to a preferred *physical* condition, and that the term *well-being* be used in speaking of the person as an *integrated whole*. What happens, then, is that the imperative placed on the other by the patient is no longer merely one of restoring the person to health, but of assisting the person in attaining well-being.

At times a "state" of well-being is not possible. For example, the person may be in a persistent vegetative state in which no physical or cognitive experience is possible because of the extensive and irreversible destruction of the neocortex. In this instance, a "condition" of well-being is the goal of those charged with the person's care. That is, the conditions that would be necessary for the attainment of a state of well-being ought to be provided even if the person is not likely to be capable of experiencing that well-being.

To accomplish this, the medical difficulty must be addressed. However, whereas when health is the goal, the elimination of the illness is the imperative; when well-being is the goal, the elimination of the suffering becomes the imperative. The moral imperative placed on the care givers is not merely one of eliminating sickness in order to restore health, nor to bring one as close as possible to what might be considered health. The imperative is one of eliminating the suffering in order that the person might enjoy well-being. In cases where suffering cannot be experienced, whatever would allow for or would generally induce suffering in that person (the condition of suffering) is to be eliminated so that the person may be in a condition of well-being.

Most often this will have to do with addressing the physical needs of the person, but it does not stop there. The moral imperative goes beyond this to include addressing the threats to wholeness brought on by the illness. That is, the imperative is not just to give an antibiotic for an infection. It is also to address the fears evoked by the person at the thought of being ill in general, or the fears that arise specifically in relation to the particular disease.

It would be helpful to recall the example of the threats to a person in illness as being illustrated by the analogy of a person tripping over a rug. When someone becomes ill, a whole series of intrarelationships (the relationships of the person with him/herself) becomes disrupted. The body image, secret life and dreams, independence, relationships with the environment, and other characteristics are upset and thrown into chaos. The body twists and turns in an attempt to regain balance. These efforts to cope may bring additional threats, additional losses of balance. The effort is to regain this balance.

The goal of care is to assist in the regaining of the balance or integrity of the person and the person's relationships with the world so that the person may live out his/her life situation in a meaningful way. To do this is to relieve or attempt to relieve the person's suffering. It needs to be made clear here that this does not ultimately depend on the success of attempts to eliminate the illness. Although certainly such an attempt needs to be made, well-being is possible even in the face of the failure of therapy.

It is true that most often well-being is served best by a return to health or to some physical state that will allow for a long and meaningful life. But

. this is not always the case. For example, some radical modification, such as an amputation, without emotional support can lead to a long and miserable life of suffering. Further, a person who is dying and being kept alive by life-sustaining interventions may also suffer terribly despite the measures being employed. Although physical life is prized as a good, and rightly so, personal integrity and well-being are greater goods.

Physical death is not an absolute evil; physical life is not an absolute value.

In the previous discussion of death, it was shown that humanity has often attempted to undue, or to at least avoid dealing with, the reality of death. Society has very often moved death into the background of existence, giving the distinct impression that death is alien to the human experience. These attitudes have a profound effect on healthcare. If death is perceived as a failure, either personal or the result of some social sin, or as some event that is not an integral part of human experience, then a fundamental healthcare goal will be to prevent death from happening. In this context, palliative care is irrational. Why would anyone seek care that allows them to be one with and bring meaning to the unfolding of their death if people are not supposed to die?

This is not an accurate understanding of death within the Judeo-Christian tradition. There is nothing, either in the Hebrew or Christian Scriptures, to suggest that physical death is not part of the nature of creation. Contemporary scholarship has suggested that a negative notion of physical death as a punishment resulting from "the fall" has been superimposed on the Scriptures by a society that fears death. Sena concludes that "God has intended death as the normal lot of humankind. . . . Death is part of God's plan; physical death cannot be avoided."[2]

The discussion of the possibility of personal reconciliation with death given in Chapter Three suggests this same conclusion. Physical death does entail a finality that makes it unique among the many and varied human experiences. That does not, however, make it foreign. Each person enjoys a physical existence that begins, develops, and comes to a close. The notion of closure may not always be a pleasant thought, but it is a mature one. It is part of the human experience to bring physical existence to closure. There is no judgment incumbent on the reality of death. The end of physical life is as natural as its beginning.

Because death is not an evil that ought not to happen, it follows that physical life is not an absolute value that must be pursued at all times. If physical death is not foreign to the human experience, then physical life may yield to what some might hold to be of greater value. For some, this might be spiritual life. This is not to say that humanity is free to abdicate physical life in favor of the spiritual. Rather, it does give insight into the fact that an acceptance of the reality that someone is dying is not tied to a defeatist attitude or to pessimism. Physical life is meant to be purposeful. The acceptance of death does not take away from that and may even facilitate it.

Häring speaks of physical life as an "exalted good, but not the only or even the highest good."[3] In fact, he writes, bodily loss in life must be able to be risked if life is to find meaning.[4] Fuchs shares this insight. He writes that although life is the fundamental value of human existence, it is not the highest value.[5] The value of physical life is not absolute.

Physical life is certainly a fundamental value, but because it is not of absolute value, it is also of relative value. By relative value I mean that its importance to a person will change over time. For someone who is young and full of promise, physical life will generally be of a great value. Life is the necessary condition, to use McCormick's words, for other values and achievements.[6] As the pursuit of further values and achievements becomes less and less possible or attractive, physical life will become of less value. This might be true of the person who is dying and coming to terms with the fact that there will not be any further physical achievements.

In a discussion of the human task, I proposed that the purpose or meaning of life is to place or discover purpose and meaning in all the moments of life. Physical life does not come prepackaged with meaning, waiting to be fulfilled according to some predetermined plan. Rather, the purpose of human physical life is to bring purpose to that physical life. Persons bring meaning to their existence. Part of that existence is the bringing to a close of physical life. It is not time that has meaning, but the human experiences that unfold during that time, whatever those experiences may be. As persons see fewer opportunities to fulfill physical potential, more physical life becomes less important. What becomes important is the meaningful living out of what is happening. As death becomes more of a reality, finding meaning in that emerges as central. When this happens, physical life must yield to physical death. The tragedy of this is found in the fact that physical death separates loved ones and brings to an end the fulfillment of possibilities, but not in the fact that it ought not to happen.

Physical death is the natural, temporal moment through which physical life, which came into existence at birth, moves beyond itself. Physical life and death are not each other's opposites. In fact, they are each other's complements. Physical life is that time when people seek to fulfill the human task of bringing meaning to the beginning and development of existence. Dying and death represent that moment when the person fulfills the human task of bringing that existence to a meaningful conclusion. There may be a belief in an afterlife. There may not be. That is not important at this point. What is important is that death, regardless of what does or does not come after it, is a time when individuals complete the human task of discovering meaning in all moments of physical existence.

This is an important conclusion, one that is influenced by, and in turn influences, the others found in this book. Every decision, every aspect of care for the ill, especially the terminally ill, will reflect one's cultural, religious, and personal attitudes toward life and death. Any exaggeration or depreciation in one's attitudes will express itself in the action called "care."

The will of the patient is fundamental for well-being.

For most people, there is the possibility, however remote, of becoming healthy when health is lost. In acute care, this is a very strong possibility. In chronic care, there is generally the possibility of attaining a condition that begins to approximate one's previous condition. This condition of physical health, however, is not primary for the person. What is primary is well-being, that is, being at one with the self in whatever health circumstances the person finds him/herself. To achieve this well-being, a person needs to be able to express his/her will in the illness. The person must exercise some control within the situation.

Throughout the preceding chapters, a constant theme that has emerged is that of *control*, of people needing to maintain or regain control within their life situation. This control is an essential part of relieving suffering, which is the sense of being out of control. No suffering can be addressed merely by the medical attention paid to a disease. Pain may be relieved, but if the fear, isolation, and changes in one's appearance or life style brought on by the disease are not addressed, the person may continue to suffer. The opportunity to exert one's own will gives the person the opportunity to exercise this control. The approach needed to relieve suffering is one that gives the person the opportunity for willful involvement in his/her own care.

The person needs to be actively involved in the healthcare decisions being made. This does not mean that the patient takes absolute responsibility for care. The medical staff does exercise a certain authority rooted in the expertise that they possess and that the person needs. Often, the medical staff knows better than the patient what needs to be done. There is also a certain authority exercised by those significant others with whom the patient shares a relationship. The person is relational, and the importance of one's relationships will exercise an influence that cannot be simply dismissed. Although it is true that the person is primary, the authority that person enjoys over the self is the authority of a person as a patient, that is, as a relational being in need.

Even so, the decision to do what needs to be done does not lie solely, or even primarily, with those who possess the expertise or with those who are inextricably linked with the person in relationships. Decisions concerning care must always reflect the will of the one who has the ultimate responsibility for living out those decisions. Without this personal authority on the part of the person, suffering can be aggravated. Taking medical charge of a patient can result in a greater sense of being out of control, causing more suffering. Likewise, decisions that ignore the person's relationships may compromise the support the person needs. Decisions, therefore, need to reflect a consensus of all the parties involved. This consensus can only be sought and found through a "trialogue" that respects the person's will, the medical profession's expertise, and the myriad of relationships involved.

The relationships that characterize this trialogue cannot be ones of subject and object. Care givers can never be subjects who, however well intentioned, manipulate an object until it is made to function in a particular way. This is especially true when the patient has chosen to function no longer, wishing to die with no further treatment. Instead, the relationships need to reflect a partnership characterized by an attitude of "doing with" the person, rather than a "doing to" or even a "doing for." The patient must, at the very least, be knowledgeable about what is happening so that, even if there is nothing active that the patient can do in the care process, the patient will still be a part of what is happening through intellectual involvement and willful assent. Only if the patient understands what is happening can he/she hope to find some meaning in it.

Beauchamp and Childress refer to this exercise of the will as the principle of autonomy.[7] They define *autonomy* as a form of personal liberty by which the person determines his/her own course of action in accordance with a plan chosen by him/herself. A person's autonomy "is his or her independence, self-reliance, and self-contained ability to decide."[8] This autonomy must be respected, and the value judgments and outlooks of the person must be recognized, even when it is believed that these judgments are mistaken. Certainly, because this person is relational, his/her plan will necessarily reflect his/her relationships. Further, because in this instance the person presents him/herself as a patient, this plan will reflect the particular needs of the person. Still, it is the person who integrates these relationships and seeks to cope with these needs. Relationships and needs will influence the exercise of autonomy, but they do not define or detract from that autonomy. Referring to Kant, Beauchamp and Childress state that respect for this autonomy is linked to the perception of the other person as having unconditional worth, simply because he/she is a person—and therefore an end in and of him/herself—determining his/her own destiny.[9]

When in the hospital, and to some degree when ill in the home, a great deal of personal independence is lost by the ill person. If the patient cannot come and go as he/she pleases, then care must allow for the freedom to be oneself in the only place he/she can be. For example, the patient should not be told not to cry because it disturbs others, whether family members, staff, or other patients. Although a patient in a hospital can be said to have a certain responsibility toward the other patients, it must also be recognized that the patient who wants and needs to cry in order to deal with what is happening has no choice but to cry where he/she is. The patient cannot go and hide in a corner. To exercise control within one's life, the person must be able to express how he/she is feeling and to cope with the crisis in which the person finds him/herself.

If the person is to truly exercise control within his/her life situation, then he/she must be free to cope, using whatever coping mechanisms are available. It is perhaps here that the true meaning of control is found. Control is not so much making all the decisions as it is making an effort to be at one with the situation by coping with it in an effective way. Control has to do with finding meaning in what is happening. The patient needs to be able to move from a sense of being attacked by illness to a sense of being ill. Although the person may not be able to fully control the process of the disease, the person can, by coping with the disease, pursue the human task of placing meaning in that illness. As this is done, the person begins to move away from seeing the self as a victim, which reinforces the sense of being out of control, toward a greater sense of responsibility for one's own being.

In this, the person seeks to "own" his/her illness, seeing illness as a part of who he/she is, rather than seeing the self as a victim of fate. This does not mean reducing the person to the illness. This should never happen, since it destroys the very core of the person. Rather, this approach views the illness as a part of who the person is as a whole being and not as something other than the person, as if a handicap has an existence unto itself and chooses to settle into a particular person. To be able to own one's situation is to be at one with it, living with it as a "part" of who the person is but never "as" who the person is. When one is able to own one's health reality, when one is able to make that health reality meaningful, then the person is well and in control, making life decisions based on who he/she is, not on what must be done because of what happened to him/her.

The patient must be able to choose to exercise or, in a given situation, to choose not to exercise control within the situation. If suffering has to do with the sense of being overwhelmed by a force over which the person has no control, and if the moral imperative is to relieve a person's suffering, then the person must be given the opportunity to exercise control within the situation by being at one with it. This is accomplished by allowing the person to participate actively in a consensus seeking trialogue that respects his/her "independence, self-reliance, and ability to decide,"[10] as well as providing the space in which the person is free to engage those coping mechanisms necessary to come to wellness in the present situation.

It should be noted that this autonomy, the exercise of the will, does not belong only to those judged competent to act. A person remains autonomous even when he/she is no longer able to deliberate and participate in the choice of a course of action. People who have become incompetent remain autonomous. Their will can be exercised in the present in accordance with its expression in the past.

In the case of Quinlan,[11] the courts determined that a respirator could be removed in lieu of her right of privacy. In subsequent cases such as Conroy and Fox, however, the courts have relied on the common law right of a person to accept or reject treatment.[12] Annas refers to this as a patient's right to self-determination,[13] a right that exists even when the patient is no longer able to make judgments. In order for a condition of well-being to exist, it is necessary that a person be able to exercise, through a proxy, his/her wishes concerning treatment, as expressed before the current crisis arose. This might be done by executing a "living will" or by appointing someone with durable power of attorney to exercise one's decision-making powers in the event of incompetence.

The patient/family is the unit of care.

Not only are the person's relationships with him/herself disrupted in illness, but the person's interrelationships are disrupted as well. The person is relational; it is part of the nature of the person to exist in relationships. When the person is ill or threatened in some way, these relationships will be affected.

All persons exist in some types of relationships, and these relationships are integrated by the person in his/her life. This is true regardless of whether the relationships are ones of intimacy or of alienation. Through changes in one's role, the prevailing cultural views concerning illness, as well as the personal views held by others, the person's relationships are changed in illness. This change can be one of abandonment and isolation on one extreme, or paternalism on the other. Ultimately the patient is left essentially alone in the face of suffering. This is especially true for people who are terminally ill. Unless these relationships are addressed, not only by assisting the patient but also by the education and support of those who are healthy, the patient's suffering will become worse. Since the person is relational, then his/her well-being is also relational. The fears and anxieties of the patient's supportive relationships must be addressed as part of the total care of the patient. Well-being is facilitated for the person when order is maintained in his/her environment.

Recall the analogy in Chapter Four of the mobile illustrating the interrelationships of the patient and family. When someone becomes ill, when part of the mobile is moved, changed, or removed, the rest of the characters are caught in a swing. Some balance needs to be restored here as well as within the life of the patient. Balance must also be regained for those who are affected by the swing brought on by another's illness. Although not ill themselves, the illness of another can be a threat that brings about suffering for them as well.

A family's emotional needs may grow as they begin to see the source of their strength or unity begin to die. Fears associated with insecurity or a loss of direction may emerge. The financial aspects of illness, especially a prolonged illness, can also be a source of tension and anxiety. The family may also experience physical needs of its own and may even require healthcare. Illness is psychosomatic, and the stress on one person brought on by another's illness can itself lead to illness. If the family is not cared for in the patient's illness, suffering will be experienced by those often thought to be the lucky ones.

In short, caring for the whole person must include care for those relationships that are integrated into the person's wholeness, as well as care for those others for whom the patient is a part of an integrated wholeness. The health of the one who is ill is not the only concern. The well-being of all those integrated into each other's lives must be the concern of those in healthcare as well.

Artificial procedures for maintaining adequate levels of nourishment and hydration are life-prolonging therapies that, as with other life-prolonging therapies, may be withheld or withdrawn when they offer the person no benefit with respect to well-being in physical living or dying.

In Chapter Four, I referred to a study by Peteet et al. showing that a patient's willingness to be nourished was influenced by emotional and psychological factors.[14] It was suggested that some patients came to identify the wasting away of their bodies, a condition known as *cachexia,* with cancer. A close look at this identification gives some insight into the ethical issue.

Identifying cachexia with the disease introduces a note of confusion. Although cachexia is a *result* of the disease, it is not *identical* with the disease. To see it as identical is to suggest that addressing the nutritional deficiency is to treat the disease. These patients believed that if they could reverse a nutritional deficiency, they would reverse the disease process. Nutrition was understood to be curative therapy, a therapy easily accepted when the person believed it would help him/her recover health. It was also noted that rigid attitudes toward eating and weight loss often reflected an unusual anxiety and feelings of helplessness over the worsening prognosis. At issue here was not really nutrition, but personal reconciliation with death.

In both these examples, the way was left open by the patient to move away from a concern to maintain adequate levels of hydration and nutrition. Emotionally, the patient ate to be cured. When the patient was able to accept the fact that cure was not possible, another reason had to be found to eat. Psychologically, the patient ate because he/she did not want to die. When the patient came to a moment of acceptance in dying, another reason had to be found to eat. In both cases, it is the state of well-being, oneness with the self as one who is going to die, that introduces the possibility that the person may no longer desire, let alone be able to tolerate, the maintenance of adequate levels of nourishment and hydration.

In addition to the emotional and psychological factors involved with this issue are the social and biological factors. People generally eat for social interaction and the support of life. As has been shown, when one comes to an acceptance of death, that person often begins to wean away from life activities as he/she brings closure to life. This involves, in many instances, moving away from some relationships. The sociability of eating may become less and less important to the person who is dying well. Also, when one is dying well, he/she is getting on with the human task of bringing life to closure. The contradiction of life-sustaining activity for the person engaged in life closure should be obvious.

Beyond the question of appetite loss, vomiting, the inability to taste, the difficulty of maintaining a nutritional balance with a progressive disease, and the fact that some patients actually die with less confusion and more comfortably without nutritional intervention at the final stages of life, is the reality that persons give meaning to their actions. When an action no longer serves the whole person, that action can become meaningless. Unless there is some personal reason to eat, as with one woman who ate scallops every day or another patient who occasionally ate popcorn even though it was not tolerated well—because they derived pleasure, not nutrition, by doing so—eating may not always be the interest of one who is approaching well-being in death.

At issue in any care for one who is ill is the well-being of that person. If eating facilitates this, then the person will eat. Most people who are terminally ill do eat, at least a little. Dying is not always easy. Closure can take a great deal of energy as the person seeks to bring the family together, makes funeral arrangements, or waits until a spouse is able to let go. Other people may want to keep up their strength for an important family or personal event. What is important to see is that each person gives meaning to his/her eating. As with all activities at this point, those that serve the interest of the patient in achieving well-being in dying are of the greatest value. The person often needs to keep his/her strength up, but not necessarily in order to prolong life. The person eats in order to have the energy he/she needs to die well.

Any intervention that *imposes* any form of care on the person is inappropriate. This includes intervention for the purpose of sustaining adequate hydration and nutrition. Peteet et al. showed that refusing to eat can be symptomatic of a need to maintain control. If it is, then this issue needs to be addressed. However, when a moving away from nutrition is a free decision based on a personal interest to do what the person is doing, that is, dying, any effort to force food or fluids will further the perception that the person has lost control. Suffering, rather than being relieved, will be aggravated.

The dying person is engaged in the human task of bringing closure to life. Any intervention with the purpose of prolonging life is contrary to the interests of the person if the person has made no request for such intervention. Certainly, most people will want to continue to eat, but at times they do not or cannot eat enough to maintain adequate fluid and nutritional levels. Artificial intervention, unless requested, is not necessarily called for, even if the person may die sooner. A cup of tea may not meet the dying person's hydrational needs, but it does have flavor, is self-administered, is more natural, and has the palliative function of moistening the mouth. This may better serve the needs of well-being.

This principle is not limited to those who are actively dying. It is not unusual for a person with a progressive terminal disease to move into and out of a semiconscious state or even lapse into a coma. Some people, as the result of some trauma, lapse into a permanent coma or a persistent vegetative state with an otherwise healthy body. In some cases such as these, a prognosis can be made with an acceptable degree of certainty that the person will not regain consciousness or resume conscious activity. For these people, it is possible to stop the human task. Their present condition makes it impossible to again pursue the human task of bringing life to growth and development. If the person is artificially maintained through some life-sustaining treatments, such as the use of respirators or through artificial hydration and nutrition, they will likewise be unable to pursue the human task of bringing physical life to closure. They are, as it were, frozen in a state of limbo.

Life is meant to be fruitful.[15] This means that life is meant to bring about the fulfillment of the human task. To keep a person in limbo, unable to do this, is to impose a condition of suffering by taking control of one's existence and not allowing any aspect of the human task to be fulfilled. Medical intervention that cannot offer the person the opportunity to move in the direction of growth and development may be withheld or withdrawn so that the person may move in the direction of closure. In order to ensure that a condition of well-being exists, it would first be necessary to determine that the person, if conscious, would not want such intervention in the given circumstances. Because the patient/family is the unit of care, it would also be necessary to ensure the understanding of loved ones.

If the person has, in the past, expressed a desire not to be maintained in a state in which the human task is frozen, then any intervention that prevents physical life from moving toward closure may be withheld or withdrawn. Closure is the direction in which the person was moving before intervention. Although intervention may be able to stop that movement, it cannot always reverse it. In such a case, medical intervention need not be continued. This will allow the person to resume the human task and bring closure to physical life.

Such a position is not without its critics. Callahan suggests that the only obstacle to such a practice is the "cluster of sentiments and emotions that is repelled by the idea of starving someone to death, even in cases where it might be for the patient's own good."[16] A similar sentiment is offered by Meilaender:

> *If we are not going to feed them because that would be nothing more than sustaining a body, why not bury them at once? No one, I think, recommends that. But if, then, they are still living beings who ought not be buried, the nourishment that all human beings need to live ought not be denied them. When we permit ourselves to think that care is useless if it preserves the life of the embodied human being without restoring cognitive capacity, we fall victim to the old delusion that we have failed if we cannot* cure *and that there is then, little point to continued* care.[17]

The Surgeon General of the United States maintains that appropriate medical care must always continue hydration and nourishment, as well as antibiotics to fight infection.[18] The state of Florida put this into law, stating in its 1984 *Life-Prolonging Procedure Act* that a listing of nonessential life-prolonging procedures "does not include the provision of sustenance or the administration of medication or performance of any medical procedure deemed necessary to provide comfort, care, or to alleviate pain."[19] Some physicians, such as Byrne, have stated that the denying of food and water is the moral equivalent of murder.[20]

Such objections notwithstanding, the position that it is morally permissible to withhold or withdraw artificial means of hydration and nourishment, as well as other forms of life-sustaining treatments, for a person who is dying or in a persistent vegetative state is not outside traditional ethical thought.[21] The contemporary objections cited seem to ignore the insights of theologians earlier in this century. Kelly and McFadden, for example, both agree that such medical intervention can be both useless and a burden to the patient.

Kelly wrote in 1950 that the use of stimulants to sustain life over a short period should be considered as ordinary medical procedures. Because they are artificial, however, and if they have little or no practical remedial value in a given circumstance, there is no obligation to use them.[22] Kelly stated further that, in the case of an incompetent person, "the patient would hardly want it." If such is the case, relatives could licitly request that it not be used.

These same arguments are applied to intravenous (IV) feeding. Kelly accepts that such intervention is in itself an ordinary practice. This does not necessarily mean, however, that it is obligatory. There are many factors that must be taken into account, including the issue of whether or not the feeding is of "any real benefit." For Kelly, the mere prolongation of physical life in some circumstances seems to be of no benefit, "and I see no sound reason for saying that the patient is obliged to submit to it."[23] With respect to patients in a coma, Kelly writes:

> *I am often asked whether such things as oxygen and intravenous feeding must be used to prolong the life of a patient, already well prepared for death, and now in a terminal coma. In my opinion, the circumstances of this case make it obvious that the non-use of artificial life-sustainers is not the same as mercy killing; and I see no reason why even the most delicate professional standard should call for their use. In fact, it seems to me that, apart from very special circumstances, the artificial means not only need not but should not be used, once the coma is reasonably diagnosed as terminal. Their use creates expense and nervous strain without conferring any real benefit.[24]*

McFadden offers similar insights into the question.[25] Writing in 1956, he admits that such interventions as IV feeding can be employed without any great inconvenience, can be called ordinary, and thus would seem to be morally compulsory procedures. His statement, however, is not absolute.

161

McFadden goes on to state that such is the case when the procedure is seen as being "temporary":

> *The above statement applies, as stated, to routine hospital cases and where the procedure is envisioned as a* temporary *means of carrying a person through a critical period. Surely any effort to sustain life permanently in this fashion would constitute grave hardship.*[26]

"Ordinary," McFadden stated, has to do with "the sound hope of benefiting the patient."[27] It would be, he adds, "ridiculous to classify any means as 'ordinary' and compulsory simply because the patient could survive it. Such a narrow concept would neither be in keeping with common sense nor moral principles."[28] Here, McFadden clearly focuses his attention on the notion of benefit. He willingly admits that offering a patient, any patient, hydration and nourishment is a common and ordinary practice, and that we are bound to feed those who are in need. He is, nevertheless, quick to point out that we are not bound to useless measures in our efforts to fulfill an affirmative duty *(nemo ad inutile tenetur)*. The intervention must offer a *real benefit* that will be enjoyed by the person for a *reasonable period of time:*

> *The fundamental principle, however, that man is not bound to the "useless" is as valid today as it ever was; and we would unhesitatingly classify an operation or course of treatment as "useless" if it does not carry with it a reasonable hope of benefiting the patient, as explained in the previous section, also a reasonable assurance that the beneficial result will be enjoyed by the patient for a worthwhile period of time.*[29]

When these facts do not exist, when there is no reasonable hope of success in giving the person any real benefit, the intervention is not morally required. To insist on the implementation of a useless procedure, a procedure that offers no remedial benefit, is to insist on a procedure that offers only an excessive burden. It is, for McFadden, that burden, flowing out of the lack of any real benefit, that constitutes the procedure as "extraordinary" and therefore not obligatory.

I have attempted to use, whenever possible, insights from the field of medicine in this work. My intention has always been to ground my reflections not in the theoretical, but in the medical reality about which I speak. For this reason, I will include medical insights in this reflection on hydration and nutrition.

The New England Journal of Medicine published in 1984 the reflections of 10 physicians on the issue of life-sustaining therapy.[30] It was their opinion that, with patients in a persistent vegetative state, it was morally permissible to withhold artificial nutrition and hydration, as well as other forms of life-sustaining treatment such as antibiotics, and to allow the person to die. It would first be necessary, however, to make a careful effort to obtain knowledge of the patient's prior wishes and to gain the understanding and agreement of the family.

The authors of the article also speak of patients who are severely and irreversibly demented; that is, people who do not initiate purposeful activity but passively accept nourishment and care. When the person's prior wishes are known, the authors state that it is morally permissible to withhold any treatment that would serve mainly to prolong dying. In cases where the person's wishes are not known, the person should receive whatever care is necessary to be kept comfortable. If the person should reject mouth feeding, it would be permissible to withhold artificial means. The authors also concluded that it is permissible to withhold treatment of an intercurrent illness. Concerning the elderly person with a permanent, yet mild, impairment of competence, the person's fluid and nutritional needs should be determined by the person's experience of thirst and hunger, not with any intention to prolong life.

These reflections are rooted in the medical reality that is present for each situation, as well as in the complications that can accompany attempts to sustain life by efforts to nourish and hydrate a person artificially. The possibility of harmful or undesirable side effects from insisting on certain levels of fluid and nutritional support have already been cited. In addition, the previous description of the different procedures for maintaining these levels, as well as the responses that accompany their implementation (such as patients pulling at their feeding tubes, thus necessitating their restraint), illustrated the burdens involved. Because intervention to maintain adequate levels of nutrition and hydration artificially may be a benefit or burden to the patient, these medical procedures are not different from other forms of life-sustaining interventions, such as the use of a respirator or dialysis in cases of end-stage renal failure. The intention of any medical intervention is to offer remedial benefit. When benefit is not possible, the procedure may be withdrawn, or even withheld. Lynn and Childress suggest three situations when hydration and nutritional support may *not* offer this benefit[31]:

1. When the procedures that would be required could be so unlikely even to restore nutritional and fluid levels to normal that they could be considered futile

2. When an improvement, although achievable, could be of no real benefit to the person, such as in the case of a persistent vegetative state and some preterminal comas
3. When the burdens to be borne outweigh the benefits to be gained.

Micetich et al. offer three conditions under which they believe the medical considerations involved would make it permissible to withdraw or withhold such intervention[32]:

1. The patient should be dying, generally within a two-week period, regardless of nutritional intervention.
2. The patient should be comatose and therefore experience no pain.
3. The family must agree that no further medical procedures need be done in the face of impending death.

Certainly a decision to withhold or withdraw artificial feeding or hydration, as with any life-sustaining treatment, is not an easy one to make. Regardless of the appropriateness of such a decision, it is nevertheless an unfortunate decision to have to make. This does not, however, make it a decision that cannot be made. A study of the withdrawal of life-sustaining treatment by Neu and Kjellstrand highlights the care that must be taken in such a decision.[33] They note, for example, the struggle of those involved in coming to the decision to withdraw life-supporting treatment:

The chart notes describing how people dealt with the problems of terminating treatment clearly showed the agony and difficulty for everyone involved. This is as it should be. If such decisions are ever made quickly or easily, patients and society should indeed worry over what goes on inside hospitals.[34]

The conclusion of their study is worthy of note:

. . . patients, physicians, and families should also be willing to consider discontinuing treatment when its main effects are only discomfort and pain. However, such a decision is obviously to be regarded as a deeply regrettable step, taken only as a last resort, at the request of the competent patient or, if the patient is incompetent, at the family's behest.[35]

The appropriateness of these decisions is supported outside the medical world as well. Public policy in the United States, as expressed in governmental studies and juridical opinions, also reflects the medical and theological position that these procedures may not always be necessary. The President's Commission for the Study of Ethical Problems in Medicine and

Biomedical and Behavioral Research, for example, states that there is no real distinction between the use of mechanical breathing devices such as respirators and mechanical feeding devices such as IV tubes. Any possible distinction, the commission suggests, seems to be based more on the emotional symbolism of providing food and water to those incapable of providing for themselves rather than on any rational difference.[36] This position is also expressed in the appellate decision of Barber, a case in which two physicians were charged with murder after removing artificial feeding from a patient.[37] The court stated that:

> *Even though these life support devices are, to a degree, "self-propelled," each pulsation of the respirator or each drop of fluid introduced into the patient's body by intravenous feeding devices is comparable to a manually administered injection or item of medication. Hence, "disconnecting" of the mechanical devices is comparable to withholding the manually administered injection or medication.*[38]

The Barber decision went on to state that medical procedures that provide hydration and nutrition are more similar to other medical procedures than to the typical human manner of eating and drinking.

In addition to the mechanics involved in artificial feeding and hydration, the President's Commission also addresses the issue of benefit. In its report, the commission defines "useless" as meaning that the continued use of a therapy cannot and does not improve the prognosis for recovery.[39] The benefit of some treatment, therefore, has to do with its ability to *improve* the situation, not merely to *maintain* it. This is not unlike McFadden's definition of "useless" as pertaining to those procedures that do not carry a reasonable assurance that the beneficial result will be enjoyed by the person for a reasonable period of time.[40]

In a further elaboration, the courts have stated that feeding, in some cases, need not be understood as being traditional treatment if it is not employed to directly cure or address the pathological condition. In some instances, the Barber decision stated, artificial feeding is meant to merely sustain biological functions in order to gain time to permit other processes to address the pathology.[41] As such, it is a therapy that could be continued indefinitely without ever actually addressing the underlying pathology. In fact, one woman lived for 37 years, 111 days, in a coma, receiving only hydration and nutritional support. Here, too, the courts seem to agree with McFadden, who stated that such procedures as artificial hydration and nutrition were intended to be a temporary means of carrying a person through a crisis.[42]

Not all juridical opinions have followed this line of reasoning. In one case, which was reversed after being appealed, the court ruled that artificial hydration and nourishment could not be withdrawn from a 48-year-old man who had entered a persistent vegetative state after undergoing surgery intended to correct an aneurysm in April 1983.[43] In its decision, the court stated that the proper focus for a decision on withdrawing life-sustaining treatment should be on the quality of the treatment furnished, not on the quality of the patient's life. The court reasoned that since the "use" of a gastrointestinal tube through which the patient was being nourished was a noninvasive, nonintrusive procedure that caused no pain or suffering, it would be inappropriate to remove it.[44] It is interesting to note here that the court recognized that, "from the aforesaid statements made by Brophy when he was competent, that his preference, if he were presently competent, would be to forego the provision of food and water by means of a G tube, and thereby terminate his life."[45] The court nevertheless made its final ruling, "irrespective of the substituted judgment of the patient."[46] The State Supreme Court later ruled in favor of the substituted judgment of the patient and allowed the removal of the gastrointestinal tube. Brophy died peacefully a few days later.

This line of reasoning is not unique to this case. In two 1987 cases involving the removal of life-sustaining intervention to maintain nutrition and hydration, the dissenting court opinions held that the focus of concern ought to be on the "objective burdens of pain and injury" caused by the treatment, as well as the expressed intent of the patient. When these objective burdens are lacking, the withdrawal of life-sustaining treatment, even with the expressed intent of the patient, is inappropriate.[47] This line of reasoning is contrary to that put forth in the President's Commission.

The President's Commission makes it clear that the notion of benefit entails more than merely the absence of some tangible burden. To be of benefit, therapy must involve some positive result.[48] This is similar to Kelly's assertion that treatment ought to have some "remedial" value.[49] If it serves no purpose, it offers no benefit. This is true regardless of the presence or absence of objective pain or intrusion. The focus should not be on the "quality" of treatment in determining if such treatment is a burden. Rather, the focus should be on the "usefulness" of the treatment. If it is useless, as defined previously, it is of no benefit. Such treatment is a burden, regardless of its noninvasive nature or use. This is also the reasoning of McFadden. With respect to the burden imposed strictly by the treatment itself, he suggested that it would be "ridiculous" to classify any means as ordinary and compulsory simply because the patient could survive it.[50] Here he repeats his contention that one is not bound to adopt useless measures in an effort to fulfill an affirmative duty. The court in the Barber case followed this line of reasoning:

> *On the other hand, a treatment course which is only minimally painful or intrusive may nonetheless be considered disproportionate to the potential benefits if the prognosis is virtually hopeless for any significant improvement in condition.*[51]

One other case I would like to cite briefly is that of a 67-year-old woman suffering from Alzheimer's disease.[52] In addition to Alzheimer's, she had suffered a stroke and was in an essentially vegetative state, being immobile, speechless, unable to swallow without choking, and barely able to cough. She also had a serious life-threatening coronary disease. Her physician recommended that if cardiac or respiratory arrest occurred, no effort should be made to attempt resuscitation. Her family agreed, but a court-appointed guardian did not.

In the Dinnerstein decision is found a definition of what it means to "prolong life":

> *'Prolongation of life' . . . does not mean mere suspension of the act of dying, but contemplates, at the very least, a remission of symptoms enabling a return towards a normal, functioning, integrated existence.*[53]

Here the court is suggesting that any treatment that cannot bring the person to a condition of well-being, as I have defined it, is merely a prolongation of *dying*, not a prolongation of *life*. The distinction is important and raises the issue of the purpose of care. The aim of care must be the bringing of the person through suffering and toward well-being. Prolonging life has to do with bringing a person out of some crisis so that he/she may resume the human task of growth and development. There is no mandate in medicine to prolong one's dying, that is, to prolong the bringing of closure to physical life. On the contrary, the obligation is to provide a condition of well-being in that closure. Prolonging it, more often than not, will merely induce a condition of suffering.

As in the literature already quoted, it is primarily the question of benefit that is the focus of contemporary theological reflections on this issue. Ramsey writes that, when someone is dying, the purpose of feeding and giving fluids is to ease and comfort the person in dying, not necessarily to preserve life.[54] The benefit that such intervention seeks to offer is one of assistance in bringing life to closure. Insofar as this intervention does this, it is appropriate. If this can be done with greater ease and comfort without nutritional intervention, then none would be required.

What of the person who is not actively dying, but instead is in a persistent vegetative state? The testimony of ethicists in court cases shows that the notion of benefit applies here as well.[55] In the case of Conroy, an elderly woman who was not able to take enough nutrition on her own, Kukura[56] testified that all procedures, surgery, or other interventions that are excessively expensive, burdensome, or inconvenient or that offer no hope of benefit to the patient are not necessary. In this particular case, he testified that the hope of recovery and of returning to cognitive life, even with nasogastric feeding, was not a reasonable possibility.[57] In this statement, Kukura seems to be making the point that the benefit must be associated with a recovery that is not incidental. Benefit must be of a certain quality.

McCormick offers some insight to this discussion by giving three possible meanings to the expression "recovery."[58] He writes that by recovery could be meant the attainment of a prior state of health, a lesser state, or a state of spontaneous vital function without consciousness. In so doing, he too, is suggesting that a recovery should be of some real significance to the person seeking it. Whereas Kelly used "remedial" and McFadden "enjoyment," McCormick uses the expression "sufficient" to indicate that a certain kind of recovery is required.[59] Using the paradigm of well-being and suffering presented in Chapter One, I will define a sufficient recovery as being that state the person can or would choose to embrace in wellness. A sufficient recovery is that recovery offering the person the possibility to pursue meaningfully the human task of growth and development in a condition of wellness. A medical treatment will be of benefit, therefore, only if it is useful in bringing about *that* recovery. When a sufficient recovery is not possible, that is, when the state of the person is such that the person cannot or would not choose for the resumption of the human task of growth and development in wellness, then the person should be allowed to move toward the task of closure, with whatever means of support are required so that well-being may be enjoyed in this. The President's Commission, which offers what are perhaps the best guidelines for addressing this issue, also suggests that one take into consideration the "extent" of recovery that can be expected in deciding whether or not a treatment is of benefit to the patient.[60]

The focus on benefit suggested here is reflected in the *Declaration on Euthanasia* and its emphasis on proportionality. The document focuses not on the quality of treatment, but on the benefit to the person *as determined by the recovery expected*. Even if the treatment involved has a noninvasive nature and use, the burden of that treatment may be in its inability to bring about a proportionate benefit. The document states this in its reaffirming of the appropriateness of stopping or refusing therapy when it falls short of expectations.[61] According to the document, this refusal is not the moral equivalent of suicide, but rather "should be seen as an acceptance of the human condition."[62]

By focusing on the human condition, the document suggests that sovereignty over life is limited, as is the obligation to prolong it. This has already been discussed in greater detail above in the principle, "Physical death is not an absolute evil; physical life is not an absolute value." The medical, legal, and theological reflections put forth here point to the fact that decisions concerning any life-sustaining procedure, including that of hydration and nutrition, must respect the limitedness that is human nature. According to the document, we are called to pursue only those procedures that will offer a proportionate benefit for the person.

I would sum up this reflection by defining what is of benefit for a patient as anything that allows the person to enjoy a condition of well-being within the pursuit of the human task. As with any other medical intervention, the maintenance of adequate levels of nutrition and hydration is to be in service to the fulfillment of this task, not undertaken for its own sake. If the quality of the nature or use of a treatment is regarded as paramount, then the human task of bringing life to closure can be disrupted, and a condition of suffering may exist. Instead, it is necessary to determine, in each case, where the person is in his/her own fulfillment of the human task and to respond with care that will assist this determination. When the task of an individual is to bring physical life to closure, suffering will result if efforts are made that delay this closure by prolonging the person's dying. When the person has begun a move toward closure, or when it is impossible to offer the person "sufficient" recovery—a recovery that offers the person the possibility to resume meaningfully the human task of growth and development—suffering may result. It is possible for medical interventions to freeze a person in a state of limbo by maintaining biological existence while at the same time, because they block any movement toward the fulfillment of the human task, disrupting personal existence.

The use of narcotics for the control of severe chronic pain is appropriate medical therapy.

Physical pain is truly an enigma. It is both necessary for biological survival and yet an experience that is often feared even more than death itself. The *Declaration on Euthanasia* states the problem this way:

> *Physical suffering is certainly an unavoidable element of the human condition; on the biological level, it constitutes a warning*

of which no one denies the usefulness; but, since it affects the human psychological makeup, it often exceeds its own biological usefulness and so can become so severe as to cause the desire to remove it at any cost.[63]

I spoke earlier of two types of pain, acute and chronic, which have little in common. Acute pain can often be treated with less difficulty. It has a transient nature that makes it predictable and easier for the person to assign it some meaning. When it arises, medication can be given to suppress it. Even when the medication is inadequate, there is a knowledge that it will eventually disappear. Chronic pain is not so easily controlled. It has a persistent nature that makes it constant and enduring. It is difficult for the person to assign chronic pain any meaning. Rather than disappear, chronic pain generally increases in intensity.

Two different types of pain, distinct in their physiological processes and in the personal experience, demand two different responses. The traditional manner of treating acute pain is to give medication as it is needed. This does not work with chronic pain because medication is always needed. Acute pain can be *relieved.* Chronic pain needs to be *prevented.* Medically, this is often done most effectively with narcotics.

The appropriateness of the use of narcotics has been the subject of discussion for some time. Pius XII addressed the issue in 1957. When asked if the suppression of pain and consciousness by the use of narcotics was permissible, even at the approach of death and if it were foreseen that their use would shorten life, he responded yes. He stipulated, however, that this was permissible only if no other means to control pain were available, and if, in the given circumstances, their use did not prevent the person from carrying out his/her religious and moral duties.[64]

Almost 25 years later, Reilly echoed the Pope's response to the issue:

Sometimes a patient's suffering is so great that it can only be alleviated by medication that is addictive or even shortens life. Although we cannot give drugs whose purpose is to end life, we can administer drugs whose secondary effect is addiction or a shorter life, provided the primary purpose is to make a patient more comfortable and better able to prepare for death.[65]

Today, the appropriateness of narcotics is still being discussed:

The fear held by physicians, nurses, patients, and family that patients will become addicted often plays a major role in the underutilization of opiate analgesics, especially of the agonists. In the terminally ill patient, consideration of a drug's addiction potential is both irrelevant and an impediment to the delivery of optimum pain relief to that patient.[66]

The cautions of which Pius XII spoke are better understood today, and the comment of McGivney and Crooks that the fears associated with their use are irrelevant can be expanded to say that they are inappropriate. Reilly's conclusion is correct, although his concern about the primary intent of the use of narcotics is overstated. Fears of drug dependence, tolerance, and addiction have been shown to be unfounded. There are no sound medical reasons not to use narcotics for the control of severe chronic pain. Reasons that are put forward are most often emotional in nature.

The emotional aspect involved in the choice of a modality of pain control highlights the need of a single patient/family unit of care. Fears on the part of the patient or the family that the patient will become a drug addict make control of pain more difficult. Both the patient and family need to be educated and helped to understand the difference between acute and chronic pain and the differences in the appropriate management of each. Both need to see that the fear of narcotics is based on the experiences of those who have abused these drugs or who have had their pain poorly managed with them in the past. This last phenomenon, poor management, occurs all too frequently:

> *In spite of the availability of an arsenal of pain medication, the underutilization of drugs for the treatment of pain, especially severe pain, is an all-too-frequent occurrence. The factors that contribute to the undermedication of patients with pain are diverse and span the fields of medicine, psychology, and sociology. . . . Proper use of currently available drugs and therapeutic modalities can provide effective pain relief for most terminally ill patients with cancer. Available treatment, however, is often inadequately applied.[67]*

Carefully titrated to the needs of the person, rather than according to a flat statistical assessment, narcotics can prevent pain from breaking through in most cases. Chronic pain can be adequately treated in no other way. By seeking to prevent pain rather than suppress it, dosage requirements are below those that would be required to induce such complications as hallucinations, somnolence, or respiratory depression.

Becoming well requires the integration of the whole person. This is not possible if the patient is preoccupied with pain or the fear of it. Well-being is also not possible if the person is drugged into a semiconscious or unconscious state. Care must be taken so that the person is able to actively participate in the human task of bringing closure to life. The *Declaration on Euthanasia* makes this same point:

> *However, painkillers that cause unconsciousness need special consideration. For a person not only has to be able to satisfy his or her moral duties and family obligations; he or she also has to prepare himself or herself with full consciousness for meeting Christ. Thus Pius XII warns: "It is not right to deprive the dying person of consciousness without a reason."*[68]

Titration of narcotics respects this obligation to keep a person free to attain well-being and prepare for salvation. In the first place, it allows for relatively small doses of the narcotic, thus allowing the person to remain alert. Secondly, by blocking pain so that it does not break through, it frees the person from the fear of future pain, a fear that would be a distraction from these same pursuits.

Used with care, narcotics offer the best hope of controlling chronic pain without the side effects often associated with their abuse. Narcotic analgesics are appropriate for the control of severe chronic pain, even when the person is expected to live over a considerable time.

Reconciliation with death is possible.

The attempts humanity has made to become reconciled with the reality of death have already been presented in some detail. My critique of these attempts showed that these were actually faulting efforts to avoid death all together, to somehow get around its reality and finality. I concluded that it seems that humanity in general cannot be truly reconciled with death, perhaps because humanity never dies in general.

A person can, however, be reconciled with his/her own death. It is possible to come to a realization that it is time to go, time to give up one's spirit. In short, it is all right to die. There is no one way to achieve this. Kübler-Ross speaks of five stages through which one might pass in order to be reconciled with death. But, as I indicated in Chapter Three by citing some critiques of her work, one does not have to go through these stages as if completing some course on dying and death. What is of value in her works and stages is that they illustrate a way to cope, a way to be reconciled with death. In doing so, they show that it is possible to achieve well-being in dying. It is possible to die well.

People often suffer when they are dying. This need not be the case. Dying is not by definition an experience that involves suffering. Death is not an ultimate evil that must be avoided; it is something that happens as part of human physical existence. Dying, the time during which one approaches death, is something people do *while they are alive.* To be dying is, by definition, to be living.

As long as someone is living, it is possible to be well in the life situation. This is accomplished through coping mechanisms that allow a person to exercise some control and discover some meaning within that situation. It is no different in death. Through coping mechanisms, people can come to terms with the fact that they are dying. Just as people might own their illness, so too can they own their dying. They move from a sense that something is killing them to a sense that they are dying. As long as something is killing the person, something coming from the outside over which there can be no control, there is suffering. However, when the person can begin to say, "I am dying," when the person can find meaning in his/her physical existence even as that existence is drawing to a close, then well-being is achieved and suffering is relieved. Kübler-Ross refers to this as acceptance.

Acceptance in well-being has nothing to do with being happy about the situation; rather, it has everything to do with being at one with a situation the person finds meaningful. One person stated openly that he was going to die and that he was "damn mad about it." There is nothing unaccepting about anger in the face of death. At the same time, there is nothing unaccepting about dying with some fear of the unknown. What is important in well-being is acceptance of the situation for what it is insofar as the person is able. It is not necessary that anyone enjoy, be happy about, or be completely at ease with the reality being accepted.

Acceptance in well-being can be tinged with denial. A person may know and inwardly accept that he/she is going to die, yet find this such a difficult reality to deal with that he/she chooses to ignore it and begins to deny it. This, too, can be a part of well-being. The person may be one with what is happening, yet choose to distance him/herself from that reality. If that is where the person chooses to be, then that is where the person is allowed to stay. The person experiences control that way. Well-being in death does not demand that one continually confront a reality that appears to be too threatening. Some people never learn to face reality in life; they cannot do this and still maintain a sense of themselves as persons. The important aspect of well-being is being at one with the situation in whatever way the person is able. Care may invite the person to move to a more active acceptance. It should, however, only invite. To force the issue would be to take control, which thus induces suffering.

Persons die in their own time.

It is the issue of well-being that suggests that people not be given a firm time line for the remainder of their life. To appear to put someone on a schedule takes away control within the dying experience and may interfere with the process of coming to terms with death. People need to be allowed to die in their own time. For one person, that might be quickly, whereas for another it may not be until the person is sure that everything has been taken care of for the survivors, or until some last-minute business, such as reconciliation with one's family or faith community, is accomplished.

In the earlier discussion of terminal illness, I noted that to be terminally ill involves not merely a disease that is by its nature terminal, but also the expectation that one will die of the effects of this disease rather than some other factors. Clinically, this is defined as being approximately six months. It needs to be stressed, however, that this is not a prediction of how much time a person has left. It is merely an indication that death is imminent. Exactly how imminent is largely up to the person dying.

Clinical evidence suggests that giving people a time frame detracts from control within the situation. Some people, when told they have six months, rally in an effort to beat the odds and to attain some final victory before death. On the one hand, this may be good for the person, giving a source of motivation for continued struggle. On the other hand, it can be asked if beating the odds is something toward which a person really wants to direct one's final efforts. When there is not much time left, spending it on things that are not all that important and that may be extremely costly in many respects might be said to be wasteful. In reality, there are no odds to beat, and living fully the time that is left seems to be preferable to getting a few more days than predicted.

Other people have been shown to lock themselves into a time frame. It is valid to question whether the medical staff is accurate in its estimates, or if people begin to prepare themselves to follow the physician's orders one more time, beginning to show deterioration or death at the time predicted. Given the difficulty in predicting the pathology of terminal illnesses, especially cancer and AIDS, the accuracy of such predictions is questionable and the power of suggestion probable.

It has also happened that patients will fully accept how little time is left and set about to prepare. Anger, disappointment, depression, and confusion can result for those who are still alive after their time is up. Clearly, being put on a schedule may detract from simply living the time that is left.

Patients are not the only ones who can suffer by this practice. Families also tend to view reality according to some frame of reference. When death is expected soon, feelings of frustration can overcome them when death does not come. Feelings of gratitude may fill some, but the difficulties and fatigue associated with having a loved one dying may cause others to wonder if the person "is ever going to die." This otherwise innocent and understandable reaction sometimes complicates the grieving process later with feelings of guilt. When predictions of some longer time are given, the family prepares to use that time to deal with some issues that need to be addressed before the person dies. If the person should die sooner than expected, feelings of grief can be complicated with a sense of being cheated or with guilt for not having acted sooner.

The practice of giving predictions can be helpful to give people a needed frame of reference. They can also be given and interpreted too literally. This may be to the detriment of the patient and the family. To achieve well-being, the person must be able to be integrated with the self as one who is dying. This must be done to the extent possible by the person in the real time available, not in an artificial time frame that may hurry some or leave others disappointed. People, to be at one with themselves in dying, must have control within the dying process. This control may be taken away when the person is told that he/she will die in a certain period. What the patient hears is not so much that "he/she will die" but that "death will come." This reinforces the notion that death is something that comes for people and that it is not possible to be reconciled with it. Suffering may be reinforced by the sense that the person has no control. It can also introduce the possibility of fear as "the date" approaches.

Although reconciliation with death is perhaps not possible for humanity in general, personal reconciliation with death is possible. Humanity will no doubt continue to fear death and seek whatever ways conceivable to get around it. The reality remains that persons who are dying can, and often do, use their coping mechanisms to come to terms with themselves as dying. This is possible when the person has the control necessary to be at one with the self, in whatever state the self happens to be. This is as true with dying as it is with having a cold. Dying well is possible.

Palliative care is an appropriate modality of care for the terminally ill.

Persons in different health situations have different healthcare needs and expectations. Some can be cured. There are, however, many who cannot be cured. To insist that healthcare must be cure oriented seems to be an injustice to the many for whom cure is not possible. This includes most of those people who have some form of cancer and perhaps all who develop AIDS. These people must be cared for in a way that addresses their specific needs. What often happens, however, is that these people get care that is oriented toward what they cannot be.

There are other people who present themselves with a need that requires some type of life-changing treatment. We may not speak of a cure per se, since the person may not be able to be cured or may not suffer from an affliction that allows for cure. A car accident, for example, is not a disease from which one is cured, but rather a situation involving injuries that may be able to be corrected to some extent. In these instances, people seek whatever changes are required in order to pursue the human task of continued growth and development. These changes may require the learning of new skills or new ways of relating; they may require a move to a new home or a change in a career. They may require the acceptance of a "new self." In all these cases, the value of physical life is high.

For other people, the value of physical life is not high, and there is little desire, energy, or possibility to implement the kinds of changes required to give more time. These people need healthcare that recognizes the futility, in whatever form futility takes, of giving more time. Having a medical approach that is principally oriented toward fostering more time seems to be an injustice to those for whom more time is not an interest.

The moral imperative is to respond to people in their suffering, not specifically to addressing the presenting need or to giving more time to life. The whole person must be helped, with the pain and grief of the present he/she carries. There is need for an approach to medical care that is not cure or time oriented simply because there are people whose health reality makes the cure impossible and time of relative value. People who cannot be cured and for whom more time is not a central interest need care that answers their particular suffering. They cannot be cared for merely by adapting the modalities of acute and chronic care to a given instance. If the moral imperative is to be fulfilled, then care must address the specific needs of these people. For them, it is the *quality of the present* that is the prime interest, not a return to what once was or more of what might be.

All care is concerned with the quality of life of the person. It must be remembered, however, that the price one is willing to pay, in terms of time, money, inconvenience, and discomfort (that is, periods of little quality), to enjoy more time, security, freedom, and comfort (periods of high quality), will change over time. It must be recognized that one may be willing to pay any price to return to a previous state or learn to live with almost any adjustment to have more time to return to what is of great importance to the person; for people who only have today, however, there is often an unwillingness to give up anything of today for a tomorrow, especially for a tomorrow that will inevitably offer less than today.

176

This does not mean that people want to die, have given up on life, or are in favor of simply doing away with anyone who is not productive in society. What it does mean is that there comes a time when the "todays" are few in number, a time when exactly how many is not nearly as important as meaningfully living however many todays there may happen to be, a time when the quality of time is a far greater value than the amount of time.

It is within this reality that the philosophy of palliative care takes its root and finds its moral justification. Palliative care responds to the moral imperative by seeking to relieve the person's suffering. This suffering that has been brought on by a disease process that the body and medical science together could not ultimately reverse, the grief from the constant loss of everything that ever seemed important, the fear of what tomorrow will bring, and the sense of abandonment by those who do not understand the disease or how the person responds to the grief and the fear it raises. In short, palliative care seeks to respond to the suffering that arises in those who perceive that fate has turned against them and who feel that they are being overwhelmed by something that is ultimately going to destroy them. Palliative care does this by allowing people control within their life and circumstances again. What was lost during the efforts to cure or prolong, palliative care seeks to return. The emphasis is on the quality of life today.

Certainly a dying person cannot control the pathology of the disease. However, control is possible in the sense that the person remains able to put order and meaning into what is happening. The dying cannot be reversed; it cannot be changed. However, how that dying unfolds and the meaning assigned to it can be controlled. In this, the person has control within the context of how he/she will die, with whom, where, and, to some extent, when. The person is also able to put meaning into the event by taking quality time to reflect and discover the meaning of one's whole life, of which this death is a part.

Palliative care focuses on the interests of the dying person. The dying person does not have an interest in becoming healthy or in living longer. The interest of the patient is to live "now." Because the person's living now involves the living out of the person's dying, there is a simultaneous interest in dying, in bringing physical life to closure. The human person has an interest in all aspects of living; in beginning it, in developing and extending it, and finally in closing it. The human task is to live out life. That "living out" takes on different meanings with time and circumstances. The goal of the human task is not so much to keep life going as to bring it to completion; that is, into existence, through growth, and to closure. Palliative care is the logical outgrowth of acute and chronic care in the pursuit of the fulfillment of this human task.

The hospitality of the palliative care unit, the emphasis on pain control, symptomatic treatment, caring for the whole person, caring for the patient and family as a single unit of care, freedom from the structures of visiting regulations, and other aspects are all in service to giving the person the opportunity to exercise control within his/her dying in order to restore the integration of wholeness that has been threatened or disrupted by the disease and efforts to treat it. The atmosphere and care are directed to giving the person what is needed to live out what is happening now.

Palliative care involves no deception. To distract anyone from the truth prevents the achievement of well-being. One cannot become one with the nonreal. Whether the truth is deliberately kept from one who is dying or implicitly denied through futile efforts to change that reality, wholeness is disrupted and dying well is prevented. The human task is blocked.

What is described here as palliative care may appear to some to be "passive euthanasia." It is not. If palliative care is to be fully appreciated, the issue of euthanasia, active or passive, must be understood.[69] The concern for a misunderstanding of palliative care as a form of euthanasia is rooted partly in a comment made by Kelly in 1950, when the ethical issues of appropriate care for the dying and the withholding and withdrawing of life-sustaining treatment were beginning to emerge. Kelly stated that the withdrawal of life support in some cases would be ethically appropriate, but that he would hesitate from publicly taking a position in a case out of fear that those who did not understand the technical distinctions involved might make reference to "a kind of Catholic euthanasia."[70] It would be unfortunate for palliative care to be understood as a "kind of euthanasia" and therefore unacceptable to many who might benefit from it.

That this misunderstanding could develop is illustrated by such work as done by Brown and Thompson. In their study of extended care facilities, they found that a decision to forego treatment of a fever in a patient is sometimes made more frequently for a person without family than for one whose family visits regularly.[71] Although the question of whether or not a fever is treated aggressively is legitimate in good healthcare, the apparent arbitrariness of the criteria by which these decisions can be made may cause some to suggest that the question itself is not legitimate and betrays an attitude that foreshadows the dangers of euthanasia.

I will approach the relationship between palliative care and euthanasia from the perspective of language, more specifically, the distinction between value and descriptive language. Bioethical and related discussions become especially difficult when language meant to describe an event is confused or associated with language that has value implications. Referring to "euthanasia" as "passive" illustrates the confusion that can arise from bringing descriptive and value language together into one expression.

First, there is difficulty with the word euthanasia itself. One of the difficulties with any discussion on euthanasia is the confusion over the precise meaning of the word. In order that there be as little confusion as possible with what I mean by palliative care, and the inappropriateness of the term euthanasia here, I will use the definitions offered by Brody[72]:

- *Euthanasia:* Intentionally expediting the death of an individual for that individual's own benefit, because of the suffering that individual is undergoing or will undergo.

- *Active euthanasia:* Euthanasia performed by means of active interventions designed to cause death directly (e.g., injecting an overdose of morphine or potassium chloride).

- *Passive euthanasia:* Euthanasia performed by means of withholding or withdrawing life-prolonging therapy (e.g., turning off a respirator or not treating a pneumonia with antibiotics).

It is sometimes argued that, in some instances of great suffering, some form of euthanasia would be an appropriate act. There are documented instances of people who have participated in another's plan to end his/her own life during an illness.[73] Accounts such as these force one to step back and recognize the limitedness of the human spirit and its desire for peace.

Even if there are some individual instances where euthanasia might be understandable, objections have been raised against a public policy that would permit such action. Dyke makes reference to the wedge principle.[74] This argument is concerned with the logic of moral justifications. To allow the practice of euthanasia as part of public policy, even in a very specific instance when it may be justified, would slowly injure society's option for life. It is not so much that some practices may actually follow as a result of such a policy, but that moral reasoning itself will be compromised. In response to calls for euthanasia, Dyke offers the Good Samaritan ideal. This approach entails a pledge not to kill one's neighbor and a commitment to be the kind of person who offers mercy and care. Such care consists of relieving pain and suffering, respecting the patient's right to refuse treatment, and providing healthcare regardless of one's ability to pay.

Foot also regards any effort to allow euthanasia as endangering the moral fiber that informs our decisions. She maintains that it may be "of the greatest importance" to keep a psychological barrier up against killing:

> *As things are, people do, by and large, expect to be looked after if they are old or ill. This is one of the good things that we have, but we might lose it, and be much worse off without it. It might come to be expected that someone likely to need a lot of looking after*

should call for the doctor and demand his own death ... in rich societies such as ours it would surely be a spiritual disaster. Such possibilities should make us very wary of supporting large measures of euthanasia, even where moral principle applied to the individual act does not rule it out.[75]

Euthanasia here is perceived as a value term in that it has an impact on moral reasoning itself. As such, it is distinct from the descriptive term *benemortasie,* or "good death." I would suggest that this distinction is found in the direct link with the "moment" of death in euthanasia, rather than with the "staying"[76] and compassion that is characteristic of care in a good death.

In palliative care there is no direct link with the moment of death. Instead, it has to do with care that allows a person to move through suffering to an acceptance of death. Palliative care is not concerned with the *when* of death, which any form of euthanasia must be concerned with because that is the intended end of one's actions with regard to the person. Palliative care is concerned with the "wellness" of death *whenever* it is lived out. To illustrate, one woman entered the palliative care unit who was expected to live only a few months. She experienced pelvic pain that was very difficult to control. Rather than dying soon, she lived for over a year and a half receiving palliative care. Any form of euthanasia, as already defined, would certainly not have "intended" that she should live so long in her condition. Palliative care allowed her to live as long as she lived. Euthanasia, in its "mercy," intends by definition to keep the dying period as short as possible. It would certainly have sought to spare her those extra months of painful dying, the same months she needed to live, and that her family and staff found difficult to endure.

Euthanasia does seek to respond to the moral imperative to relieve suffering. It does this, however, by eliminating the person who is suffering. As such, euthanasia contradicts everything put forth concerning the meaning of the person, well-being, and suffering. To put another out of misery by taking or deliberately shortening that person's life denies the fundamental value of physical life and grows out of an attitude, however understandable, of pessimism. Requests for euthanasia in patients who are suffering from a painful, progressive disease very often flow from pessimism, desperation, and despair. Saunders (personal communication) maintains that when people ask for euthanasia, what they are really seeking is relief from pain.

Life can have meaning, and because dying is a part of life, it also can have meaning, but only if the person places or discovers it there. To choose to die through some medical intervention is to deny the human task, which includes allowing physical life to come to closure. Choosing euthanasia or engaging in an act of suicide is to give up, rather than seek acceptance in, well-being. It is to abdicate control in life to another person or to a disease, thus limiting the possibility of achieving well-being. Such an attitude could be the result of poor medical care that has not allowed the person the opportunity to achieve well-being and put meaning into his/her suffering, or a fear of suffering born out of some past experience or the suffering of others. It may also grow out of a life that itself has seemed meaningless. Certainly if one has not been able to find meaning in life, he/she may not expect that it could be found in death.

To choose to practice euthanasia on others is to take over for oneself another's human task of bringing that life to closure. Just as someone cannot live out the life of another, someone also cannot bring another's life to closure. The one who practices euthanasia may not know the real needs or the fears and anxieties of the person dying. The person may lie quietly in bed, but this may be the effect of the drugs, not the well-being of the person. Suffering may not be relieved at all. The person may very well die in a condition of suffering, the very suffering that was thought to be relieved. Suffering remains because the person has indeed been overwhelmed by an outside force over which he/she has no control. The destruction of the person that was feared is now accomplished. I should emphasize that it is not my place or intention to judge other people's actions or intentions. My point, however, is that situations in which people choose or participate in acts of euthanasia are tragic because they are unnecessary. There is, I believe, a better way to die.

Palliative care is not euthanasia. The purpose of palliative care is to allow the person to bring life to closure, to own one's own dying and die well. There is no intention to do that work for the person. Palliative care does not seek to simply eliminate suffering. Rather, it seeks to allow the person to give meaning to that suffering and move toward well-being.

Finally, there is a difficulty with the word *passive,* which might be said to qualify the value term euthanasia and make it morally acceptable. Passive is a descriptive term; it describes one's relationship to something. As a descriptive term, it is entirely inappropriate in this context. Palliative care is not passive at all. Palliative care is *active* care.

Palliative care cannot be equated with passive care or simple hand-holding. Although hands should be and are held, palliative care seeks to relieve the suffering of the person. This entails caring for the whole person in an environment that offers security, hope, and welcome. As I have already described in some detail, it is exercised by an interdisciplinary team with expertise in all aspects of care. Care only appears to be passive. This is sometimes because pain is being so well controlled, through an accurate assessment of the person's total pain and the appropriate titration of narcotic analgesics, that an air of unhurried calm pervades the palliative care unit. Yet the attention given to all aspects of the patient's well-being rules out any merely passive or "do nothing" attitude. True, nothing is done necessarily to prolong the person's dying, but a great deal is done to assist in the living out of that dying.

CONCLUSION

These final ethical principles of healthcare are my conclusions. This final section is simply an attempt to summarize this book.

The person is an integration of many different characteristics. The uniqueness of each person is reflected in these characteristics—in their presence and intensity, their root and influence, and the way they are integrated into oneness. Each person is engaged in life in fulfilling the human task, that is, of integrating these characteristics into a oneness through a beginning, a development, and a closing of physical life. Many of life's elements may threaten this wholeness. This work has been concerned with the threats involved in illness. Illness threatens the integrity of a person by causing changes in the characteristics that make up that person. When these change, one's balance is lost and integration must again be achieved. When it is, that person is well.

At times in life, the person may feel overwhelmed by these threats. A sense may grow that the person is out of control and going to be overwhelmed by some force. Ultimately, it is believed this force will destroy the person. More than the fear of death itself is this fear of being destroyed. This experience I call suffering.

Responding to the moral imperative to relieve the suffering of others is the task of all people. This entails addressing not only the immediate needs of the person, but also assisting that person to regain the wholeness or integration that has been lost. This effort is to assist the person in moving from a condition of suffering to a condition of well-being. This does not depend on bringing the person from illness to health, although that may be a major part of the process.

It is part of the human task to bring physical life to closure so that life itself may come to fulfillment. The process of dying is threatening to the person. It involves fears, anxieties, and grief beyond those brought on by illness. The person's integrity is threatened, and suffering becomes part of the dying experience. The person seeks to relieve his/her own suffering by exercising some control within his/her life. In dying, the person may engage in denial, expressions of anger, acts of bargaining, and/or periods of depression. All this is an effort to cope with the impending death. If efforts to become once again an integrated and whole person succeed, even as he/she dies, and if the person can place or discover meaning in what is happening and be at one with him/herself as one who is dying, then the person can move through suffering and be well—not healthy perhaps, but well.

People often need assistance in this task. When someone presents him/herself to another as one who is suffering in the act of dying, the moral imperative is to relieve that suffering. This is done by assisting the person to come to accept, although not necessarily like, the reality of death. Palliative care seeks to do this by pursuing a mode of care that gives the person control within his/her own dying. This is done through medical intervention that is symptomatic as well as offering psychosocial and spiritual support to the patient and to the family, who is also intimately involved in the dying of the patient. The effort is always to give the person the highest quality of life that this person can enjoy today. By giving the person the opportunity to stop looking for the impossible cure or to keep living as long as possible with no hope of improvement, the person becomes free to find oneness with the self again and to die well.

NOTES

1. For a discussion of the relationship between the Judeo-Christian tradition and North American ethical thought, see Robert M. Veatch, *A Theory of Medical Ethics,* Basic Books, New York, 1981; especially Chapter 2, "The Dominant Western Competitors: The Judeo-Christian Tradition," pp. 27-42. See also Richard A. McCormick, "Theology and Biomedical Ethics," *Église et Théologie* 13, 1982, pp. 311-331.
2. Patrick J. Sena, "Biblical Teaching on Life and Death," in *Moral Responsibility in Prolonging Life Decisions,* eds. Donald G. McCarthy and Albert S. Moraczewski, Pope John XXIII Medical-Moral Research & Education Center, St. Louis, 1981, p. 17 (hence referred to as *Moral Responsibility*).
3. Bernard Häring, *Medical Ethics,* Fides Publishers, Notre Dame, IN, 1973, pp. 66 and 68.
4. Häring, p. 69.
5. Joseph Fuchs, "Control over Human Life? Bioethical Questions Today," *Theology Digest* 32, 1985, pp. 247-252.
6. Richard A. McCormick, *How Brave a New World: Dilemmas in Bioethics,* Doubleday & Co., Garden City, NY, 1981, p. 395.
7. Tom L. Beauchamp and James F. Childress, *Principles of Biomedical Ethics,* Oxford University Press, New York, 1979, pp. 56-96.
8. Beauchamp and Childress, p. 56.

9. Beauchamp and Childress, pp. 58-59.
10. Beauchamp and Childress, p. 56.
11. *In the Matter of Karen Quinlan,* 70 NJ 10 355 A.2d 647 (1976).
12. *In the Matter of Claire Conroy,* 486 A.2d 1209 1985 (NJ 1985); and *In the Matter of Philip K. Eichner, S.M., On Behalf of Brother Joseph C. Fox v. Dillon,* 420 North Eastern Reporter 2d Series 1980, p. 64.
13. George J. Annas, "When Procedures Limit Rights: From Quinlan to Conroy," *The Hastings Center Report* 15, 1985, pp. 24-26.
14. John R. Peteet et al., "Psychological Aspects of Artificial Feeding in Cancer Patients," *Journal of Parenteral and Enteral Nutrition* 5, 1981, pp. 138-140.
15. Sacred Congregation for the Doctrine of the Faith, *Declaration on Euthanasia,* U.S. Catholic Conference, Washington, DC, 1980, p. 4.
16. Daniel Callahan, "On Feeding the Dying," *The Hastings Center Report* 13, 1983, p. 22.
17. Gilbert Meilaender, "On Removing Food and Water: Against the Stream," *The Hastings Center Report* 14, 1984, pp. 11-13. See also his essay "Caring for the Permanently Unconscious Patient," in *By No Extraordinary Means,* ed. Joanne Lynn, Indiana University Press, Bloomington, 1986, pp. 195-201.
18. John J. Paris and Andrew C. Varga, "Care of the Hopelessly Ill," *America,* Sept. 22, 1984, p. 143.
19. See Florida Code, chapter 765, section 765.03. This statute was cited in an August 1985 Florida trial court decision that denied a man's request to remove a feeding tube from his 78-year-old wife who had been in a persistent vegetative state for three years. See "Feeding: Treatment or Care?" *Ethical Currents* 5, 1985, p. 5.
20. Paris and Varga, p. 143, quoting Dr. Paul Byrne as saying, "Denying food and water to such patients is murder," *USA Today,* March 29, 1984.
21. For a history of the Catholic moral teaching on prolonging life issues, see Gary M. Atkinson, "Theological History of Catholic Teaching on Prolonging Life," in *Moral Responsibility,* pp. 95-115; and James J. McCartney, "The Development of the Doctrine of Ordinary and Extraordinary Means of Preserving Life in Catholic Moral Theology Before the Karen Quinlan Case," *Linacre Quarterly* 47, 1980, pp. 215-237.
22. Gerald Kelly, "The Duty of Using Artificial Means of Preserving Life," *Theological Studies* 11, 1950, p. 218.
23. Kelly, p. 219.
24. Kelly, p. 220.
25. Charles J. McFadden, *Medical Ethics,* 4th ed., F.A. Davis, Philadelpia, 1956.
26. McFadden, p. 270.
27. McFadden, p. 267.
28. McFadden, p. 282.
29. McFadden, p. 282.
30. Sidney H. Wanzer et al., "The Physician's Responsibility Toward Hopelessly Ill Patients," *The New England Journal of Medicine* 310, 1984, pp. 955-959.
31. Joanne Lynn and James F. Childress, "Must Patients Always Be Given Food and Water?" *The Hastings Center Report* 13, 1983, pp. 17-21.

32. Kenneth Micetich, Patricia Steinecker, and David Thomasma, "Are Intravenous Fluids Morally Required for a Dying Patient?" *Archives of Internal Medicine* 143, 1983, pp. 975-978.
33. Steven Neu and Carl M. Kjellstrand, "Stopping Long-Term Dialysis: An Empirical Study of Withdrawal of Life-Supporting Treatment," *The New England Journal of Medicine* 314, 1986, pp. 14-20.
34. Neu and Kjellstrand, p. 19.
35. Neu and Kjellstrand, p. 19.
36. President's Commission for the Study of Ethical Problems in Medicine and Biomedical and Behavioral Research, *Deciding to Forego Life-Sustaining Treatment: A Report on the Ethical, Medical, and Legal Issues in Treatment Decisions,* U.S. Government Printing Office, Washington, DC, 1983, p. 192, footnote 52.
37. It is estimated that at least six physicians in the United States have been accused of murder for withdrawing or withholding life-supporting treatment in recent years. See Neu and Kjellstrand, p. 14.
38. *Barber v. Superior Court of California,* 195 Cal. Rptr. 484C Cal. App. 2 Dist. 1983, p. 1017, section 9. See also Bonnie Steinbock, "The Removal of Mr. Herbert's Feeding Tube," *The Hastings Center Report* 13, 1983, pp. 13-16.
39. President's Commission, p. 191, footnote 50, quoting Dennis Horan, "Euthanasia and Brain Death: Ethical and Legal Considerations," *Annals NY Academy of Science* 315, 1978, pp. 363-367.
40. McFadden, p. 282.
41. *Barber,* p. 1020, section 11.
42. McFadden, p. 270.
43. *Brophy v. New England Sinai Hospital, Inc.,* Commonwealth of Massachusetts, The Probate and Family Court Department, Docket No. 85E0009-G1.
44. *Brophy,* p. 42.
45. *Brophy,* p. 25.
46. *Brophy,* p. 42.
47. See NJ Sup. Ct.: *In re Peter,* No. A-78, 6/24/87, and NJ Sup. Ct.: *In re Jobes,* No. A-108, 6/24/87, in *The United States LAW WEEK* 56, LW2021.
48. President's Commission, pp. 82-90.
49. Kelly, p. 218.
50. McFadden, p. 282.
51. *Barber,* p. 1020, section 11.
52. *In the Matter of Shirley Dinnerstein,* 380 N.E. 2d 134 (Mass. App. Ct. 1978).
53. *Shirley Dinnerstein,* p. 38.
54. Paul Ramsey, *The Patient as Person: Explorations in Medical Ethics,* Yale University Press, New Haven, CT, 1970, pp. 128-129.
55. For an insightful article on the role of ethicists in the courts, see Peter G. McAllen and Richard Delgado, "Moral Experts in the Courtroom," *The Hastings Center Report* 14, 1984, pp. 27-34.
56. Joseph Kukura is a Roman Catholic priest and an associate professor of Christian Ethics at the Immaculate Conception Seminary, Mahwah, NJ.
57. *Conroy,* p. 1218.
58. McCormick, p. 388.

59. McCormick, p. 388.
60. President's Commission, p. 88.
61. *Declaration on Euthanasia,* p. 10.
62. *Declaration on Euthanasia,* pp. 10-11.
63. *Declaration on Euthanasia,* p. 7.
64. Pius XII, "Allocutio" *AAS* 49, 1957, pp. 129-147, p. 147. See also Pius XII, "Allocutiones," *AAS* 50, 1958, p. 687-700, p. 694-695.
65. Lawrence T. Reilly, "Prolonging Life Conscience Formation," in *Moral Responsibility,* p. 144.
66. William T. McGivney and Glenna M. Crooks, "The Care of Patients with Seveve Chronic Pain in Termial Illness," *Journal of the American Medical Association* 251, 1984, pp. 1182-1188.
67. McGivney and Crooks, p. 1182.
68. *Declaration on Euthanasia,* p. 8.
69. John F. Tuohey, "Hospice Care and Passive Euthanasia: Can They Be Equated?" *The American Journal of Hospice Care* 4, 1987, pp. 30-33.
70. Kelly, p. 219.
71. Norman K. Brown and Donovan J. Thompson, "Non-treatment of Fever in Extended Care Facilities," *The New England Journal of Medicine* 300, 1979, pp. 1246-1250.
72. Howard Brody, *Ethical Decisions in Medicine,* 2nd ed., Little, Brown & Co., Boston, 1981, p. 232, section 789.
73. See Betty Rollin, *Last Wish,* Linden Press/Simon & Shuster, New York, 1985; recounts the story of a woman's struggle to respond to her 66-year-old mother's request for assistance in hastening her death of cancer. In another case, on Jan. 20, 1986, a young man in a Phoenix, AZ, hospital pulled the plug on his brother's life support system and held off police for two hours with a shotgun. The brother survived, and police considered charging the young man with attempted murder.
74. Arthur Dyke, "The Good Samaritan Ideal and Beneficent Euthanasia: Conflicting Views of Mercy," *Linacre Quarterly* 42, 1975, pp. 176-188.
75. Philippa Foot, "Euthanasia," in *Intervention and Reflection: Basic Issues in Medical Ethics,* 2nd ed., ed. Ronald Munson, Wadsworth Publishing Company, Belmont, CA, 1983, pp. 163-174.
76. Jeanne Q. Benoliel and Dorothy M. Crowley, *The Patient in Pain: New Concepts,* American Cancer Society, New York, 1974, p. 7.

Bibliography

"Acquired Immune Deficiency Syndrome (AIDS): Precautions for Clinical and Laboratory Staffs," *Morbidity and Mortality Weekly Report* 32, 1983, pp. 450-451.

Ajemian, Ina, "General Principles of Symptomatic Management," in *The R.V.H. Manual on Palliative/Hospice Care,* eds. Ina Ajemian and Balfour M. Mount, Ayer Company Publishers, Salem, NH, 1982, pp. 184-199.

Aldrich, C. Knight, "Some Dynamics of Anticipatory Grief," in *Anticipatory Grief,* eds. Bernard Schoenberg, Arthur C. Carr, Austin H. Kutscher, et al., Columbia University Press, New York, 1974, pp. 3-9.

Angell, Marcia, "Disease as a Reflection of the Psyche," *The New England Journal of Medicine* 312, 1985, pp. 1570-1572.

Annas, George J., "When Procedures Limit Rights: From Quinlan to Conroy," *The Hastings Center Report* 15, 1985, pp. 24-26.

Ariès, Philippe, "Five Variations on Four Themes," in *Death: Current Perspectives,* 3rd ed., ed. Edwin S. Shneidman, Mayfield Publishing, Palo Alto, CA, 1984, pp. 62-72.

Ashley, Benedict M., "An Integrated Christian View of the Human Person," in *Technological Powers and the Person,* eds. Albert S. Moraczewski, Donald G. McCarthy, Edward J. Bayer, et al., Pope John XXIII Medical-Moral Research & Education Center, St. Louis, 1983, pp. 313-333.

Ashley, Benedict M., and O'Rourke, Kevin D., eds., *Health Care Ethics: A Theological Analysis,* 2nd ed., The Catholic Health Association of the United States, St. Louis, 1982.

Atkinson, Gary M., "Theological History of Catholic Teaching on Prolonging Life," in *Moral Responsibility in Prolonging Life Decisions,* eds. Donald G. McCarthy and Albert S. Moraczewski, Pope John XXIII Medical-Moral Research & Education Center, St. Louis, 1981, pp. 95-115.

Bader, Diana, and McMillan, Elizabeth, *AIDS: Ethical Guidelines for Healthcare Providers,* The Catholic Heath Association of the United States, St. Louis, 1987.

Baines, Mary B., "Principles of Symptom Control," in *The R.V.H. Manual on Palliative/Hospice Care,* eds. Ina Ajemian and Balfour M. Mount, Ayer Company Publishers, Salem, NH, 1982, pp. 176-183.

Bakan, David, *Disease, Pain and Sacrifice: Toward a Psychology of Suffering,* Beacon Press, Chicago, 1971.

Barber v. Superior Court of California, 195 Cal. Rptr. 484C Cal. App. 2 Dist. 1983.

Barbour, Stephen David, "Acquired Immunodeficiency Syndrome of Childhood," *Pediatric Clinics of North America* 34, 1987, pp. 247-268.

Barnes, Deborah M., "AIDS Commission Bills Proliferate," *Science* 235, 1987, p. 1136.

Barnes, Deborah M., "Brain Damage by AIDS Under Active Study," *Science* 235, 1987, pp. 1574-1577.

Bates, Thelma D., "Radiotherapy in Terminal Care," in *The Management of Terminal Disease,* ed. Cicely M. Saunders, Edward Arnold Publishers Ltd., London, 1978, pp. 119-124.

Bates, Thelma D., and Vanier, Thérèse, "Palliation by Cytotoxic Chemotherapy and Hormone Therapy," in *The Management of Terminal Disease,* ed. Cicely M. Saunders, Edward Arnold Publishers Ltd., London, 1978, pp. 125-133.

Bean, Glynis, Cooper, Sloan, Alpert, Renee, and Kipnis, David, "Coping Mechanisms of Cancer Patients: A Study of 33 Patients Receiving Chemotherapy," *CA—A Cancer Journal for Clinicians* 30, 1980, pp. 256-259.

Beauchamp, Tom L., and Childress, James F., *Principles of Biomedical Ethics,* Oxford University Press, New York, 1979.

Beauchamp, Tom L., and McCullough, Laurence B., *Medical Ethics: The Moral Responsibilities of Physicians,* Prentice-Hall, Englewood Cliffs, NJ, 1984.

Becker, Ernest, "The Terror of Death," in *Death: Current Perspectives,* 3rd ed., ed. Edwin S. Shneidman, Mayfield Publishing, Palo Alto, CA, 1984, pp. 62-72.

Benoliel, Jeanne Q., and Crowley, Dorothy M., *The Patient in Pain: New Concepts,* American Cancer Society, New York, 1974.

Berger, Joseph R., "Neurologic Complications of Human Immunodeficiency Virus Infection: What Diagnostic Features to Look for," *Postgraduate Medicine* 81, 1987, pp. 72-77.

Blaney, Robert L., and Piccola, Gary E., "Psychologic Issues Related to AIDS," *Journal of the Medical Association of Georgia* 76, 1987, pp. 28-32.

Blum, Henrik L., *Planning for Health: Development and Application of Social Change,* Behavioral Publishers, New York, 1974.

Blumberg, Eugene M., "Results of Psychological Testing of Cancer Patients," in *The Psychological Variables in Human Cancer,* eds. Joseph A. Gengerelli and Frank J. Kirkner, University of California Press, Berkeley, 1954, pp. 30-61.

Blumberg, Eugene M., West, Philip M., and Ellis, Frank W., "MMPI Findings in Human Cancer," in *Basic Readings on the MMPI in Psychology and Medicine,* eds. George Schlager Welsh and W. Grant Dahlstrom, University of Minnesota Press, Minneapolis, 1956, pp. 452-460.

Blumberg, Eugene, M., West, Philip M., and Ellis, Frank W., "A Possible Relationship Between Psychological Factors and Human Cancer," *Psychosomatic Medicine* 16, 1954, pp. 277-286.

Blumenfield, Michael, Smith, Peggy Hordano, and Milazzo, Jane, "Survey of Nurses Working with AIDS Patients," *General Hospital Psychiatry* 9, 1987, pp. 58-63.

Bonica, John J., "Cancer Pain," in *The R.V.H. Manual on Palliative/Hospice Care,* eds. Ina Ajemian and Balfour M. Mount, Ayer Company Publishers, Salem, NH, 1982, pp. 113-144.

Bonica, John J., "Importance of the Problem," in *Advances in Pain Research and Therapy,* vol. 2, eds. John J. Bonica, Vittorio Ventafridda, B. Raymond Fink, et al., Raven Press, New York, 1979, pp. 1-12.

Borgelt, Bruce B., Geleer, Richard, Kramer, Simon, et al., "The Palliation of Brain Metastases: Final Results of the First Two Studies by the Radiation Therapy Oncology Group," *International Journal of Radiation Oncology, Biology & Physics* 6, 1980, pp. 1-9.

Boyd, Peggy, *The Silent Wound: A Startling Report on Breast Cancer and Sexuality,* Addison-Wesley, Reading, MA, 1984.

Brady, Luther W., "The Changing Role of Radiation Oncology in Cancer Management," *Cancer* 51, 1983, pp. 2506-2514.

Brody, Howard, *Ethical Decisions in Medicine,* 2nd ed., Little, Brown & Co., Boston, 1981.

Brophy v. New England Sinai Hospital, Inc., Commonwealth of Massachusetts, The Probate and Family Court Department, Docket No. 85E0009-G1.

Brown, Norman K., and Thompson, Donovan J., "Non-treatment of Fever in Extended Care Facilities," *The New England Journal of Medicine* 300, 1979, pp. 1246-1250.

Buckley, Jerry, and Gelman, David, "Living with Cancer," *Newsweek,* April 8, 1985, pp. 64-71.

Cady, Blake, Simpson, Howard N., Farrish, Grover, and Turner, John W., "History Taking for Cancer Detection," in *Cancer: A Manual for Practitioners,* 5th ed., ed. Blake Cady, American Cancer Society, Boston, 1978, pp. 1-12.

Callahan, Daniel, "On Feeding the Dying," *The Hastings Center Report* 13, 1983, p. 22.

Calman, K.C., "Physical Aspects," in *The Management of Terminal Disease,* ed. Cicely M. Saunders, Edward Arnold Publishers Ltd., London, 1978, pp. 33-43.

Campbell, Alastair V., *Professional Care: Its Meaning and Practice,* Fortress Press, Philadelphia, 1984.

"Can a Nurse be Fired for Having AIDS?" *American Dental Association News,* 1987, pp. 3, 9.

Cancer: A Manual for Practitioners, 5th ed., ed. Blake Cady, American Cancer Society, Boston, 1978.

"Candidate AIDS Vaccine," *Science* 235, 1987, p. 1575.

Carter, R.L., "Pathological Aspects," in *The Management of Terminal Disease,* ed. Cicely M. Saunders, Edward Arnold Publishers Ltd., London, 1978, pp. 19-32.

Cassel, Eric J., "The Nature of Suffering and the Goals of Medicine," *The New England Journal of Medicine* 306, 1982, pp. 630-645.

Cassidy, Judy, "Withholding or Withdrawing Nutrition and Fluids: What Are the Real Issues? An Interview with Reverend John J. Paris," *Health Progress,* December 1985, pp. 22-25.

Cassileth, Barrie R., Luck, Edward J., et al., "Psychosocial Correlates of Survival in Advanced Malignant Disease?" *The New England Journal of Medicine* 312, 1985, pp. 1551-1555.

Centers for Disease Control, "Recommendations for Prevention of HIV Transmission in Health-Care Settings," *Morbidity and Mortality Weekly Report* 36, 1987, pp. 1s-18s.

Clark, Gregory L., and Vinters, Harry V., "Dementia and Ataxia in a Patient with AIDS," *The Western Journal of Medicine* 1, 1987, pp. 68-72.

Clark, Matt, Morris, Holly, King, Patricia, et al., "Learning to Survive," *Newsweek,* April 8, 1985, pp. 72-77.

Clark, Tim, "Man at the Crossroads," *Yankee,* May 1984, pp. 70-73, 166-169.

Cohen, Sidney, "Marijuana, Does It Have a Possible Therapeutic Use?" *Journal of the American Medical Association* 240, 1978, pp. 1761-1763.

Coil, James H., III, "Legal Issues Involving AIDS," *Journal of the Medical Association of Georgia* 76, 1987, pp. 64-68.

Cooper, Jay S., and Fried, Peter R., "Defining the role of radiation therapy in the management of Epidemic Kaposi's Sarcoma," *International Journal of Radiation Oncology, Biology & Physics* 13, 1987, 35-39.

Cooperband, Sidney R., "Immunology: Overview and Future Prospects," in *Cancer: A Manual for Practitioners,* 5th ed., ed. Blake Cady, American Cancer Society, Boston, 1978, pp. 71-79.

Coping with Cancer: A Resource for the Health Professional, U.S. Department of Health and Human Services, National Cancer Institute, NIH pub. no. 80-2080, Bethesda, MD, September, 1980.

Corbeil, Madeleine, "Nursing Process for a Patient with a Body Image Disturbance," *Nursing Clinics of North America* 6, 1971, pp. 155-163.

Cousins, Norman, *Anatomy of an Illness as Perceived by the Patient: Reflections on Healing and Regeneration,* Bantam Books, New York, 1979.

Craven, Joan, and Wald, Florence S., "Hospice Care for Dying Patients," *American Journal of Nursing* 75, 1975, pp. 1816-1822.

Curran, James W., Morgan, Meade, Hardy, Ann M., et al., "The Epidemiology of AIDS: Current Status and Future Prospects," *Science* 229, 1985, pp. 1352-1357.

"D.C., 21 States Bar AIDS Discrimination. Disease Victims Considered 'Handicapped' by Law," *American Dental Association News* 3, 1987, pp. 1, 3.

de la Peña, Augustin M., *The Psychobiology of Cancer: Automatization and Boredom in Health and Disease,* Bergin Publishers, South Hadley, MA, 1983.

Death: Current Perspectives, 3rd ed., ed. Edwin S. Shneidman, Mayfield Publishing, Palo Alto, CA, 1984.

Death and Society: A Book of Readings and Sources, eds. James P. Carse and Arlene B. Dallery, Harcourt Brace Jovanovich, New York, 1977.

Deckers, Peter J., McDonough, Eugene F., Jr., and Shipley, William U., "The Physical Examination for Cancer Detection," in *Cancer: A Manual for Practitioners,* 5th ed., ed. Blake Cady, American Cancer Society, Boston, 1978, pp. 13-17.

Derogatis, Leonard R., Abeloff, Martin D., and Melisaratos, Nick, "Psychological Coping Mechanisms and Survival Time in Metastatic Breast Cancer," *Journal of the American Medical Association* 242, 1979, pp. 1504-1508.

Devita, Vincent T., Jr., Broder, Samuel, Fauci, Anthony, et al., "Developmental Therapeutics and the Acquired Immunodeficiency Syndrome," *Annals of Internal Medicine* 106, 1987, pp. 568-581.

"Does a Terminal Patient Have a Right to Die?" A poll of nurses conducted by *Nursing Life,* in *Good Housekeeping,* May 1984, pp. 81-84.

Douglas, Carolyn J., and Druss, Richard G., "Denial of Illness: A Reappraisal," *General Hospital Psychiatry* 9, 1987, pp. 53-57.

Dunphy, J. Englebert, "Annual Discourse: On Caring for the Patient with Cancer," in *Cancer: A Manual for Practitioners,* 5th ed., ed. Blake Cady, American Cancer Society, Boston, 1978, pp. 337-350.

Dyke, Arthur, "The Good Samaritan Ideal and Beneficent Euthanasia: Conflicting Views of Mercy," *Linacre Quarterly* 42, 1975, pp. 176-188.

Endean, Eric D., Ross, Charles W., and Strodel, William E., "Kaposi's Sarcoma Appearing as a Rectal Ulcer," *Surgery* 101, 1987, pp. 767-769.

Evan, Elida A., *A Psychological Study of Cancer,* Dodd, Mead & Co., New York, 1926.

Evans, Jocelyn, *Living with a Man Who is Dying: A Personal Memoire,* Taplinger Publishing, New York, 1971.

Eyre, Harmon J., "Advances in Cancer Management," in *Proceedings of the National Conference on Practice, Education, and Research in Oncology Social Work—1984,* American Cancer Society, Boston, 1984, pp. 1-4.

Farr, William C., "Should Heroin Be Available for Pain?" *Journal of the American Medical Association* 241, 1979, pp. 882-883.

"Feeding: Treatment or Care?" *Ethical Currents,* November 1985, no. 5, p. 5.

Feigenberg, Loma, *Terminal Care: Friendship Contracts with Dying Cancer Patients,* trans. Patrick Hort, Brunner/Mazel, New York, 1980.

Fischl, Margaret A., Richman, Douglas, Grieco, Michael H., et al., and the AZT Collaborative Working Group, "The Efficacy of Azidothymidine (AZT) in the Treatment of Patients with AIDS and AIDS-Related Complex," *The New England Journal of Medicine* 317, 1987, pp. 185-191.

Fisher, Margaret C., "Transfusion-Associated Acquired Immunodeficiency Syndrome—What Is the Risk?" *Pediatrics* 79, 1987, pp. 157-160.

Fletcher, Joseph, "Indicators of Humanhood: A Tentative Profile of Man," *The Hastings Center Report* 2, 1972, pp. 1-4.

Foot, Philippa, "Euthanasia," in *Intervention and Reflection: Basic Issues in Medical Ethics,* 2nd ed., ed. Ronald Munson, Wadsworth Publishing Co., Belmont, CA, 1983, pp. 163-174.

Freymann, John G., *The American Health Care System: Its Genesis and Trajectory,* Med Communications Publications, New York, 1974.

Frierson, Robert L., and Lippmann, Steven B., "Psychologic Implications of AIDS," *American Family Physician* 35, 1987, pp. 109-116.

Fuchs, Joseph, "Control over Human Life? Bioethical Questions Today," *Theology Digest* 32, 1985, pp. 247-252.

Gallo, Robert C., "The AIDS Virus," *Science* 235, 1987, pp. 46-56.

Gates, Christopher C., "Psychological Issues in Cancer," in *Cancer: A Manual for Practitioners,* 5th ed., ed. Blake Cady, American Cancer Society, Boston, 1978, pp. 80-90.

Glick, John H., "Palliative Chemotherapy: Risk/Benefit Ratio," in *Clinical Care of the Terminal Cancer Patient,* eds. Barrie R. Cassileth and Peter A. Cassileth, Lea & Febiger, Philadelphia, 1982, pp. 53-63.

Gorer, Geoffrey, "The Pornography of Death," in *Death: Current Perspectives,* 3rd ed., ed. Edwin S. Shneidman, Mayfield Publishing, Palo Alto, CA, 1984, pp. 26-30.

Gostin, Larry, and Curran, William J., "Legal Control Measures for AIDS: Reporting Requirements, Surveillance, Quarantine, and Regulation of Public Meeting Places," *The American Journal of Public Health* 77, 1987, pp. 214-218.

Green, Elmer, and Green, Alyce, *Beyond Biofeedback,* Delacorte Press, New York, 1977.

Griffiths, Bede, "Hinduism," in *New Catholic Encyclopedia,* vol. VI, ed. William S. McDonald, McGraw-Hill, New York, 1967, pp. 1123-1136.

Grisez, Germain G., and Boyle, Joseph M., Jr., *Life and Death with Liberty and Justice: A Contribution to the Euthanasia Debate,* University of Notre Dame Press, Notre Dame, IN, 1979.

Häring, Bernard, *Medical Ethics,* Fides Publishers, Notre Dame, IN, 1973.

Harnish, Delsworth G., Hammerberg, Ole, Walker, Irwin R., and Rosenthal, Kenneth L., "Early Detection of HIV Infection in a Newborn," *The New England Journal of Medicine* 316, 1987, pp. 272-273.

Henderson, Nancy, "Supreme Court Reverses AIDS Judgment," *Nature* 326, 1987, p. 115.

Hetzel, Paul C., Hoovis, Marvin L., and Kaufman, Sheldon D., "Overall Principles of Cancer Management. IV. Chemotherapy," in *Cancer: A Manual for Practitioners,* 5th ed., ed. Blake Cady, American Cancer Society, Boston, 1978, pp. 59-67.

Hilgartner, Margaret W., "AIDS and Hemophilia," *The New England Journal of Medicine* 317, 1987, pp. 1153-1154.

Himes, Michael, "The Human Person in Contemporary Theologies: From Human Nature to Authentic Subjectivity," in *Technological Powers and the Person,* eds. Albert S. Moraczewski, Donald G. McCarthy, Edward J. Bayer, et al., Pope John XXIII Medical-Moral Research & Education Center, St. Louis, 1983, pp. 288-312.

Hirsch, Martin S., Wormser, Gary P., Schooley, Robert T., et al., "Acquired Immunodeficiency Syndrome," *Annals of Internal Medicine* 104, 1986, pp. 575-581.

Hollander, Harry, "Practical Management of Common AIDS-Related Medical Problems," *Western Journal of Medicine* 146, 1987, pp. 137-240.

Holmes, Sarah W., and Peel, Jesse, "Meeting the Mental Health Challenge of AIDS and Related Disorders," *Journal of the Medical Association of Georgia* 76, 1987, pp. 33-34.

Hoskisson, J. Bradley, *Loneliness: an Explanation, a Cure,* Citadel Press, New York, 1965.

In the Matter of Claire Conroy, 486 A.2d 1209 1985 (NJ 1985).

In the Matter of Karen Quinlan, 70 NJ 10 355 A.2d 647 (1976).

In the Matter of Philip K. Eichner, S.M., On Behalf of Brother Joseph C. Fox v. Dillon, 420 North Eastern Reporter 2d Series 1980, p. 64.

In the Matter of Shirley Dinnerstein, 380 N.E. 2d 134 (Mass. App. Ct. 1978).

Jackson, David L., and Younger, Stuart, "Patient Autonomy and 'Death with Dignity': Some Clinical Caveats," *The New England Journal of Medicine* 301, 1979, pp. 404-408.

Janssens, Louis, "Artificial Insemination: Ethical Considerations," *Louvain Studies* 8, 1980, pp. 3-29.

Janssens, Louis, "Norms and Priorities in a Love Ethic," *Louvain Studies* 6, 1977, pp. 207-238.

Janssens, Louis, "Personalist Morals," *Louvain Studies* 3, 1970, pp. 5-16.

Jaroff, Leon, "Can Attitude Affect Cancer?" *Time,* June 24, 1985, p. 69.

Kastenbaum, Robert J., *Death, Society, and Human Experience,* 3rd ed., The C.V. Mosby Co., St. Louis, 1985.

Keen, Lisa M., "A Personal Experience with AIDS," *The American Journal of Hospice Care* 3, 1986, pp. 10-16.

Kelly, Gerald, "The Duty of Using Artificial Means of Preserving Life," *Theological Studies* 11, 1950, pp. 203-220.

Klein, Robert S., Phelan, Joan A., Freeman, Katherine, et al., "Low Occupational Risk of Human Immunodeficiency Virus Infection Among Dental Professionals," *The New England Journal of Medicine* 318, 1988, pp. 86-90.

Krant, Melvin J., "What Cancer Means to Society," in *Proceedings of the American Cancer Society Third National Conference on Human Values and Cancer,* American Cancer Society, Washington, DC, 1981, pp. 15-19.

Kübler-Ross, Elisabeth, *Death: The Final Stage of Growth,* Prentice-Hall, Englewood Cliffs, NJ, 1975.

Kübler-Ross, Elisabeth, *Living with Death and Dying,* Macmillan, New York, 1981.

Kübler-Ross, Elisabeth, *On Death and Dying,* Macmillan, New York, 1969.

Kübler-Ross, Elisabeth, *Questions and Answers on Death and Dying,* Macmillan, New York, 1974.

Kübler-Ross, Elisabeth, "What is it like to be dying?" *The American Journal of Nursing* 71, 1971, pp. 54-61.

Lazarus, Richard S., "Positive Denial: The Case for Not Facing Reality," *Psychology Today* 13, 1979, pp. 44-60.

LeShan, Lawrence L., *You Can Fight for Your Life: Emotional Factors in the Causation of Cancer,* M. Evans & Co., New York, 1977.

Levene, Martin B., "Overall Principles of Cancer Management. III. Radiation Therapy," in *Cancer: A Manual for Practitioners,* 5th ed., ed. Blake Cady, American Cancer Society, Boston, 1978, pp. 49-58.

Levine, Stephen, *Who Dies? An Investigation of Conscious Living and Conscious Dying,* Anchor Press/Doubleday & Co., Garden City, NY, 1982.

Li, Frederick P., Hall, Deborah J., and McDonald, Jill A., "Cancer Epidemiology, Risk Factors, and Screening," in *Cancer: A Manual for Practitioners,* 5th ed., ed. Blake Cady, American Cancer Society, Boston, 1978, pp. 22-29.

Lifton, Robert J., and Olson, Eric, *Living and Dying,* Bantam Books, New York, 1974.

Lipman, Arthur G., "Drug Therapy in Cancer Pain," *Cancer Nursing* 3, 1980, pp. 39-46.

Los Angeles County–University of Southern California Cancer Center, *Psychological Aspects of Cancer,* LAC–USC Publication, Los Angeles, 1983.

Loscalzo, Matthew, "Pain and Anxiety Control," in *Proceedings of the National Conference on Practice, Education, and Research in Oncology Social Work—1984,* American Cancer Society, 1984, pp. 22-25.

Lynn, Joanne, and Childress, James F., "Must Patients Always Be Given Food and Water?" *The Hastings Center Report* 13, 1983, pp. 17-21.

The Management of Terminal Disease, ed. Cicely M. Saunders, Edward Arnold Publishers Ltd., London, 1978.

The Many Faces of AIDS: A Gospel Response, United States Catholic Conference, Washington, DC, 1987.

Markel, William M., and Sinon, Virginia, "The Hospice Concept," in *American Cancer Society Professional Education Publication,* American Cancer Society, Boston, 1978.

Marmor, Michael, Friedman-Kein, Alvin E., Zolla-Pazner, Susan, et al., "Kaposi's Sarcoma in Homosexual Men," *Annals of Internal Medicine* 100, 1984, pp. 809-815.

Maslow, Abraham H., *Toward a Psychology of Being,* 2nd ed., Van Nostrand Publishers, Princeton, NJ 1968.

Matthews, Gene W., and Neslund, Verla, "The Initial Impact of AIDS on Public Health Law in the United States—1986," *Journal of the American Medical Association* 257, 1987, pp. 344-352.

May, William F., "Institutions as Symbols of Death," in *Death and Society: A Book of Readings and Sources,* eds. James P. Carse and Arlene B. Dallery, Harcourt Brace Jovanovich, New York, 1977, pp. 407-426.

Mayer, Kenneth H., and Opal, Steven M., "Therapeutic Approaches for AIDS and HIV Infection," *Rhode Island Medical Journal* 70, 1987, pp. 27-33.

McAllen, Peter G., and Delgado, Richard, "Moral Experts in the Courtroom," *The Hastings Center Report* 14, 1984, pp. 27-34.

McCartney, James J., "The Development of the Doctrine of Ordinary and Extraordinary Means of Preserving Life in Catholic Moral Theology Before the Karen Quinlan Case," *Linacre Quarterly* 47, 1980, pp. 215-237.

McCormick, Richard A., *How Brave a New World: Dilemmas in Bioethics,* Doubleday & Co., Garden City, NY, 1981.

McCormick, Richard A., *Notes on Moral Theology: 1965 Through 1980,* University Press of America, Washington, DC, 1981.

McCormick, Richard A., "Notes on Moral Theology: 1983," *Theological Studies* 45, 1984, pp. 80-138.

McCormick, Richard A., "Theology and Biomedical Ethics," *Église et Théologie* 13, 1982, pp. 311-331.

McFadden, Charles J., *Medical Ethics,* 4th ed., F.A. Davis, Philadelphia, 1956.

McGill, Arthur C., *Suffering: A Test of Theological Method,* Westminster Press, Philadelphia, 1982.

McGivney, William T., and Crooks, Glenna M., "The Care of Patients with Severe Chronic Pain in Terminal Illness," *Journal of the American Medical Association* 251, 1984, pp. 1182-1188.

Meilaender, Gilbert, "On Removing Food and Water: Against the Stream," *The Hastings Center Report* 14, 1984, pp. 11-13.

Meissner, William A., "Pathologic Evaluation and Classification of Tumors," in *Cancer: A Manual for Practitioners,* 5th ed., ed. Blake Cady, American Cancer Society, Boston, 1978, pp. 30-38.

Melzack, Ronald, "Current Concepts of Pain," in *The R.V.H. Manual on Palliative/Hospice Care,* eds. Ina Ajemian and Balfour M. Mount, Ayer Company Publishers, Salem, NH, 1982, pp. 96-112.

Micetich, Kenneth, Steinecker, Patricia, and Thomasma, David, "Are Intravenous Fluids Morally Required for a Dying Patient?" *Archives of Internal Medicine* 143, 1983, pp. 975-978.

Mount, Balfour M., "Correspondence: a letter to the editor of the *CMA Journal*," reprinted in *The R.V.H. Manual on Palliative/Hospice Care,* eds. Ina Ajemian and Balfour M. Mount, Ayer Company Publishers, Salem, NH, 1982, pp. 165-166.

Mount, Balfour M., "Introduction to Death and Dying Services in the Acute Care Hospital" (keynote address), delivered at the Fourth International Seminar on Terminal Care, Montreal, Canada, 1983.

Mount, Balfour M., "Narcotic Analgesics in the Treatment of Pain of Advanced Malignant Disease," in *The R.V.H. Manual on Palliative/Hospice Care,* eds. Ina Ajemian and Balfour M. Mount, Ayer Company Publishers, Salem, NH, 1982, pp. 148-164.

Mount, Balfour M., Ajemian, Ina, and Scott, J.F., "Use of the Brompton Mixture in Treating the Chronic Pain of Malignant Disease," *CMA Journal* 115, 1976, pp. 122-124.

Mozden, Peter J., and Cady, Blake, "Overall Principles of Cancer Management. V. Hormone Therapy," in *Cancer: A Manual for Practitioners,* 5th ed., ed. Blake Cady, American Cancer Society, Boston, 1978, pp. 68-70.

Munley, Anne, *The Hospice Alternative: A New Context for Death and Dying,* Basic Books, New York, 1983.

Myers, W.P. Laird, "Attitudes of Physicians as Revealed in Their Approaches to Patients with Advanced Cancer," in *Proceedings of the American Cancer Society Third National Conference on Human Values and Cancer,* American Cancer Society, Washington, DC, 1981, pp. 59-68.

National Center for Health Statistics, "AIDS Myths," *Newsweek,* Nov. 16, 1987, p. 6.

Nelson, James B., and Rohricht, Jo Anne Smith, *Human Medicine: Ethical Perspectives on Today's Medical Issues,* rev. ed., Augsburg Publishing House, Minneapolis, 1984.

Neu, Steven, and Kjellstrand, Carl M., "Stopping Long-Term Dialysis: An Empirical Study of Withdrawal of Life-Supporting Treatment," *The New England Journal of Medicine* 314, 1986, pp. 14-20.

Nisbet, Robert, "Death," in *Death: Current Perspectives,* 3rd ed., ed. Edwin S. Shneidman, Mayfield Publishing, Palo Alto, CA, 1984, pp. 119-122.

Nobler, Myron P., Leddy, Mary Ellen, and Huh, Sun H., "The Impact of Palliative Irradiation on the Management of Patients with Acquired Immune Deficiency Syndrome," *Journal of Clinical Oncology* 5, 1987, pp. 107-112.

Norris, Catherine, "Body Image: Its Relevance to Professional Nursing," in *Behavioral Concepts and Nursing Intervention,* 2nd ed., eds. Carolyn E. Carlson and Betty Blackwell, J.C. Lippincott, Philadelphia, 1978, pp. 5-36.

Oswei, Tempkin, "Health and Disease," in *Dictionary of the History of Ideas,* vol. 2, ed. Philip P. Weiner, Charles Scribner's Sons, New York, 1973, pp. 395-407.

Oswei, Tempkin, "The Scientific Approach of Disease: Specific Entity and Individual Sickness," in *Scientific Changes,* ed. Alistair C. Crombie, Heinemann, London, 1963, pp. 629-660.

Pace, Omar T., and Cady, Blake, "Overall Principles of Cancer Management. II. Surgery," in *Cancer: A Manual for Practitioners,* 5th ed., ed. Blake Cady, American Cancer Society, Boston, 1978, pp. 43-48.

"Pain Terms: A List with Definitions and Notes on Usage," recommended by the International Association for the Study of Pain, Subcommittee on Taxonomy, *Pain* 6, 1979, pp. 249-252.

Paris, John J., and Varga, Andrew C., "Care of the Hopelessly Ill," *America,* Sept. 22, 1984, pp. 141-144.

Parkes, C. Murray, "Psychological Aspects," in *The Management of Terminal Disease,* ed. Cicely M. Saunders, Edward Arnold Publishers Ltd., London, 1978, pp. 44-64.

Pepper, Curtis B., "The Victors: Patients Who Conquered Cancer," *New York Times Magazine,* Jan. 29, 1984, pp. 14-20, 24-28.

Peteet, John R., Medeiros, Cynthia, Slavin, Leslie, and Walsh-Burke, Katherine, "Psychological Aspects of Artificial Feeding in Cancer Patients," *Journal of Parenteral and Enteral Nutrition* 5, 1981, pp. 138-140.

Pius XII, "Adstantibus multis honorbilibus Viris ac praeclaris Medicis et Studiosis, quorum plerique Nosocomiis praesunt vel in magnis Lyceis docent, qui Roman convenerant invitatu et arcessitu Instituti Genetici 'Gregoirio Mendel' Summus Pontifex propositis quaesitis de 'reanimatione' respondit," *Acta Apostolicae Sedis—Commentarium Officiale* 49, 1957, pp. 1027-1033.

Pius XII, "Allocutio," *Acta Apostolicae Sedis—Commentarium Officiale* 49, 1957, pp. 129-147.

Pius XII, "Allocutiones," *Acta Apostolicae Sedis—Commentarium Officiale* 50, 1958, pp. 687-700.

Prescott, David M., and Flexer, Abraham S., *Cancer: The Misguided Cell,* Sinauer Associates, Sunderland, MA, 1982.

President's Commission for the Study of Ethical Problems in Medicine and Biomedical and Behavioral Research, *Deciding to Forego Life-Sustaining Treatment: A Report on the Ethical, Medical, and Legal Issues in Treatment Decisions,* U.S. Government Printing Office, Washington, DC, 1983.

Proceedings of the American Cancer Society Third National Conference on Human Values and Cancer, American Cancer Society, Washington, DC, 1984.

Ramsey, Paul, *The Patient as Person: Explorations in Medical Ethics,* Yale University Press, New Haven, 1970.

Reichert, Cheryl M., O'Leary, Timothy J., Levens, David L., et al., "Autopsy Pathology in the Acquired Immune Deficiency Syndrome," *American Journal of Pathology* 112, 1983, pp. 357-382.

Reidy, Maurice, *Foundations for a Medical Ethic: A Personal and Theological Exploration of the Ethical Issues in Medicine Today,* Veritas Publications, Dublin, 1978.

Reilly, Lawrence T., "Prolonging Life Conscience Formation," in *Moral Responsibility in Prolonging Life Decisions,* eds. Donald G. McCarthy and Albert S. Moraczewski, Pope John XXIII Medical-Moral Research & Education Center, St. Louis, 1981, pp. 139-146.

Richter, Melvyn P., "Palliative Radiation Therapy," in *Clinical Care of the Terminal Cancer Patient,* eds. Barrie R. Cassileth and Peter A. Cassileth, Lea & Febiger, Philadelphia, 1982, pp. 65-75.

Ries, J., "Manichaeism," in *New Catholic Encyclopedia,* vol. IX, ed. William S. McDonald, McGraw-Hill, New York, 1967, pp. 153-160.

Roberts, Sharon L., *Behavioral Concepts and the Critically Ill Patient,* Prentice-Hall, Englewood Cliffs, NJ, 1976.

Robertson, John A., *The Rights of the Critically Ill,* Bantam Books, New York, 1983.

Robinson, Gene, Wilson, Samuel E., and Williams, Russel A., "Surgery in Patients with Acquired Immunodeficiency Syndrome," *Archives of Surgery* 122, 1987, pp. 170-175.

Rollin, Betty, *Last Wish,* Linden Press/Simon & Schuster, New York, 1985.

Rosenberg, Steven A., "Combined-Modality Therapy of Cancer: What Is It and When Does It Work?" *The New England Journal of Medicine* 312, 1985, pp. 1512-1514.

Rosenberg, Steven A., Lotze, Michael T., Muul, Linda M., et al., "Observations on the Systemic Administration of Autologous Lymphokine-Activated Killer Cells and Recombinant Interleukin-2 to Patients with Metastatic Cancer," *The New England Journal of Medicine* 313, 1985, pp. 1485-1492.

Sacred Congregation for the Doctrine of the Faith, *Declaration on Euthanasia,* U.S. Catholic Conference, Washington, DC, 1980.

Sanford, John A., *Evil: The Shadow Side of Reality,* Crossroad Publishing, New York, 1981.

Saunders, Cicely M., "Appropriate Treatment, Appropriate Death," in *The Management of Terminal Disease,* ed. Cicely M. Saunders, Edward Arnold Publishers Ltd., London, 1978, pp. 1-9.

Saunders, Cicely M., "Patient Care: An Introduction," in *Topics in Therapeutics,* ed. D.W. Vere, Pitman Press, London, 1978, pp. 72-110.

Schoen, Kitsy, "Psychological Aspects of Hospice Care for AIDS Patients," *The American Journal of Hospice Care* 3, 1986, pp. 35-37.

Schotsmans, Paul, "Decision Making and Personal Conscience in Medical Care," unpublished paper, 1984.

Schulz, Richard, and Aderman, David, "Clinical Research and the Stages of Dying," *Omega* 5, 1974, pp. 137-143.

Scitovsky, A.A., and Rice, D.P., "Estimates of the Direct and Indirect Costs of Acquired Immunodeficiency in the United States, 1985, 1986, and 1991," *Public Health Report* 102, 1987, pp. 5-17.

Sena, Patrick J., "Bibical Teaching on Life and Death," in *Moral Responsibility in Prolonging Life Decisions,* eds. Donald G. McCarthy and Albert S. Moraczewski, Pope John XXIII Medical-Moral Research & Education Center, St. Louis, 1981, pp. 3-19.

Shneidman, Edwin S., "Some Aspects of Psychotherapy in Dying Persons," in *Death: Current Perspectives,* 3rd ed., ed. Edwin S. Shneidman, Mayfield Publishing, Palo Alto, CA, 1984, pp. 272-283.

Showalter, J. Stuart, and Andrew, Brian L., *To Treat or Not to Treat: A Working Document for Making Critical Life Decisions,* The Catholic Health Association of the United States, St. Louis, 1984.

Simonton, O. Carl, Matthews-Simonton, Stephanie, and Creighton, James L., *Getting Well Again: A Step-by-Step Self-Help Guide to Overcoming Cancer for Patients and Their Families,* Bantam Books, New York, 1978.

Sourkes, Barbara M., *The Deepening Shade: Psychological Aspects of Life-Threatening Illness,* University of Pittsburgh Press, Pittsburgh, 1982.

Spiers, Alexander S.D., "The Palliative Management of Cancer Patients," in *Cancer: A Manual for Practitioners,* 5th ed., ed. Blake Cady, American Cancer Society, Boston, 1978, pp. 307-316.

Steinbock, Bonnie, "The Removal of Mr. Herbert's Feeding Tube," *The Hastings Center Report* 13, 1983, pp. 13-16.

Stoddard, Sandol, *The Hospice Movement: A Better Way of Caring for the Dying,* Jonathan Cape, London, 1978.

Strauss, Anselm L., *Chronic Illness and the Quality of Life,* The C.V. Mosby Co., St. Louis, 1984.

Sunderland, Ronald H., and Shelp, Earl E., *AIDS: A Manual for Pastoral Care,* The Westminster Press, Philadelphia, 1987.

Sunderland, Ronald H., and Shelp, Earl E., *AIDS and the Church,* The Westminster Press, Philadelphia, 1987.

"Surgeon General's Report on Acquired Immune Deficiency Syndrome," *Journal of the Medical Association of Georgia* 76, 1987, pp. 48-54.

Sylvester, Edward, *Target: Cancer,* Charles Scribner's Sons, New York, 1986.

Taylor, Phyllis B., "Understanding Sexuality in the Dying Patient," *Nursing '83* 13, 1983, pp. 54-55.

Taylor, Rick, "Cancer Patients Face Prejudice on Job," *Springfield (MA) Sunday Republican,* Nov. 25, 1984, sec. II, p. B1.

Temple of the Holy Spirit: Sickness and Death of the Christian in the Liturgy, the Twenty-First Liturgical Conference Saint Serge, trans. Matthew J. O'Connell, Pueblo Publishing, New York, 1975.

Thompson, Leslie M., "Dealing with AIDS and Fear: Would You Accept Cookies From an AIDS Patient?" *Southern Medical Journal* 80, 1987, pp. 228-232.

Tillich, Paul, "The Meaning of Health," in *Religion and Medicine,* ed. David R. Belgum, Iowa State University Press, Ames, IA, 1967, pp. 3-12.

Toynbee, Arnold, "The Relation Between Life and Death, Living and Dying," in *Death: Current Perspectives,* 3rd ed., ed. Edwin S. Shneidman, Mayfield Publishing, Palo Alto, CA, 1984, pp. 8-14.

Toynbee, Arnold, "Various Ways in Which Human Beings Have Sought to Reconcile Themselves to the Fact of Death," in *Death: Current Perspectives,* 3rd ed., ed. Edwin S. Shneidman, Mayfield Publishing, Palo Alto, CA, 1984, pp. 73-96.

Trent, Bill, "AIDS Has Created a New Form of Bereavement," *California Medical Association Journal* 136, 1987, p. 194.

Tsongas, Paul, *Heading Home,* Alfred A. Knopf, New York, 1984.

Tsoukas, Chris, "AIDS: Future Implications for Palliative Care," *Journal of Palliative Care* 21, 1986, pp. 35-38.

Tuazon, Carmelita U., and Labriola, Ann M., "Management of Infectious and Immunological Complications of Acquired Immunodeficiency Syndrome (AIDS): Current and Future Prospects," *Drugs* 33, 1987, pp. 66-84.

Tuohey, John F., "Hospice Care and Passive Euthanasia: Can They Be Equated?" *The American Journal of Hospice Care* 4, 1987, pp. 30-33.

Tuohey, John F., "Palliative Care," *New Catholic World* 230, 1987, pp. 187-191.

Twycross, Robert G., "Clinical Experience with Diamorphine in Advanced Malignant Disease," *International Journal of Clinical Pharmacology, Therapy and Toxicology* 7, 1974, pp. 197-198.

Twycross, Robert G., "Relief of Pain," in *The Management of Terminal Disease,* ed. Cicely M. Saunders, Edward Arnold Publishers Ltd., London, 1978, pp. 65-98.

Veatch, Robert M., *A Theory of Medical Ethics,* Basic Books, New York, 1981.

Wall, Patrick D., "On the Relation of Injury to Pain," *Pain* 6, 1979, pp. 253-264.

Wanzer, Sidney H., Adelstein, S. James, Cranford, Ronald E., et al., "The Physician's Responsibility Toward Hopelessly Ill Patients," *The New England Journal of Medicine* 310, 1984, pp. 955-959.

Weil, Andrew, *Health and Healing: Understanding Conventional and Alternative Medicine,* Houghton Mifflin, Boston, 1983.

Weisman, Avery D., "Common Fallacies About Dying Patients," in *Death: Current Perspectives,* 3rd ed., ed. Edwin S. Shneidman, Mayfield Publishing, Palo Alto, CA, 1984, pp. 222-225.

Weisman, Avery D., *On Dying and Denying: A Psychiatric Study of Terminality,* Behavioral Publications, New York, 1972.

Whalen, James P., "Participation of Medical Students in the Care of Patients with AIDS," *Journal of Medical Education* 62, 1987, pp. 53-54.

Williams, Michael R., "The Place of Surgery in Terminal Care," in *The Management of Terminal Care,* ed. Cicely M. Saunders, Edward Arnold Publishers Ltd., London, 1978, pp. 134-138.

Williamson, John B., *Aging and Society,* Holt, Rinehart & Winston, New York, 1980.

Wood, William C., and Binder, Sheldon C., "Biopsy Principles," in *Cancer: A Manual for Practitioners,* 5th ed., ed. Blake Cady, American Cancer Society, Boston, 1978, pp. 18-21.

Worden, William J., "Teaching Adaptive Coping to Cancer Patients," in *Proceedings of the American Cancer Society Third National Conference on Human Values and Cancer,* American Cancer Society, Washington, DC, 1981, pp. 129-138.

Wormer, Gary, Joline, Carol, Duncanson, Frederick, and Cunningham-Rundles, Susanna, "Needlestick Injuries During the Care of Patients with AIDS," *The New England Journal of Medicine* 310, 1984, p. 1461.

Wortman, Camille B., and Dunkell-Schetter, Christine, "Interpersonal Relationships and Cancer: A Theoretical Analysis," *Journal of Social Issues* 35, 1979, pp. 120-155.

Zerwekh, Joyce V., "The Dehydration Question," *Nursing '83* 13, 1983, pp. 47-51.

Zorza, Victor, and Zorza, Rosemary, *A Way to Die,* Alfred A. Knopf, New York, 1980.

Index

ARC. *See* AIDS-related complex
  (ARC)
Ashley, Benedict M., 15
Asymptomatic infection, 32
Autonomy, 154
Autopsy, 28
Azidothymidine (AZT), 115
AZT. *See* Azidothymidine (AZT)
Barber, 165, 167
Bargaining, 69, 71
Barnes, Deborah M., 116
Beam irradiation, 104
Bean, Glynis, 42, 43
Beauchamp, Tom L., 154
Benemortasie, 180
Benoliel, Jeanne Q., 118, 124
Biofeedback, 13-14
Biological health, 10
Blaney, Robert L., 43
Blood, and AIDS, 29
Body, 5-6, 33-37, 63
Body image, 5-6, 33-37
Bonica, John J., 123, 124, 125
Boyd, Peggy, 26
Brahma, 13
Brands, Paul, 117
Brody, Howard, 179
Brompton's Cocktail, 133
Brophy, 166
Brown, Norman K., 178
Buddhism, 63
Byrne, Paul, 161
Cachexia, 157
Callahan, Daniel, 160
Cancer
  current data, xi
  definition and cause, 24-26
  metastatic, 27-28
  nature of, 24-28
  and pain, 118
  and therapies, 101-12
  as threat to person, 32-51
  warning signs, 24

Carcinoma, 27
Care
  ethical principles of, 148-82
  modalities of, 85-86
  morally responsible, 147-86
  palliative. *See* Palliative care
  and relationships, 156-57
Cassel, Eric J., 2, 3, 4, 5, 7, 18
Cassileth, Barrie R., 26
CDC. *See* Centers for Disease
  Control (CDC)
Centeredness, self-. *See* Self-
  centeredness
Centers for Disease Control
  (CDC), 28-29, 30, 115
Central nervous system (CNS), 14,
  28
Character, and personality, 3
Chemical health, 10
Chemotherapy, 28, 37, 38, 52,
  108-12, 115
  aggressive, 108-11
  and AIDS, 115
  palliative, 111-12
Childress, James F., 138, 154, 163
Christianity, 63
Christian tradition, 2, 13, 149, 151
Chronic care, 85-86
Chronic pain, 121-22, 123, 169-72
CKS. *See* Classic Kaposi's sarcoma
  (CKS)
Clark, Gregory L., 116
Classic Kaposi's sarcoma (CKS),
  98, 113
  See also Epidemic Kaposi's
    sarcoma (EKS) *and*
    Kaposi's sarcoma (KS)
Clinically advanced phase, of
  tumor growth, 26-27
Clinically early phase, of tumor
  growth, 26
CNS. *See* Central nervous system
  (CNS)

Esteem. *See* Self-esteem
Ethical principles, of care for
    terminally ill, 148-82
Euphoriant Solution, 133
Euthanasia, 62, 168, 169-70, 172,
    178, 179, 180-81
  active and passive, 179
Evan, Elida A., 25
Event, and pain, 121
Falwell, Jerry, 13
Family, and patient, 156-57
Fatigue, 120
FDA. *See* Food and Drug
    Administration (FDA)
Fear, 120
Feldman, 47
Fight-or-flight response, 121
Fischl, Margaret A., 115
Fisher, Margaret C., 30
Food and Drug Administration
    (FDA), 113
Foot, Philippa, 179
Fox, Joseph C., 156
Fried, Peter R., 114
Frierson, Robert L., 35, 39
Fuchs, Joseph, 152
Future, and person, 3
Galen, 25
Gendron, 25
Generalized lymphadenopathy, 32
Genesis, 62, 63
Glick, John H., 111
Gliomas, 28
Good Samaritan, 63, 179
Gorer, Geoffrey, 64
Green, Alyce, 14
Green, Elmer, 14
Grief, 72, 77
Growth fraction, 109
Guilt, 36, 71
Häring, Bernard, 2, 152

Health, 149
  characterists of, 10
  defined, 9-12
  paradigm of, 15-20
  and sickness, 9-15
Healthcare, modalities of, 85-86
Hedonism, 62
Hemophilia, 50
Hepatitis, 44
Heroin, 133
Heterosexuality. *See* Sexuality
Hinduism, 13
Historical health, 10
HIV. *See* Human
    immunodeficiency virus
    (HIV)
Hodgkin's disease, 102, 106, 108,
    110
Homosexuality. *See* Sexuality
Hopelessness, internal, 33
Hoskisson, J. Bradley, 41
Hospice Mix, 133
HTLV-III. *See* Human T-
    lymphotropic virus type III
    (HTLV-III)
Human condition, 169
Human immunodeficiency virus
    (HIV), 29, 30, 36, 44, 46, 48,
    49, 50, 112, 115, 116, 117
  classification, 32
  replication cycle, 31-32
Human T-lymphotropic virus type
    III (HTLV-III), 29, 44, 112
Hurt, and pain, 119-20
Illness
  perspectives on, 12-14
  terminal. *See* Terminal illness
Image, body, 5-6, 33-37
Independence, 37-39
Infections, 32
  opportunistic, 115-17

The Catholic Health Association of the United States is the national organization of Catholic hospitals and long term care facilities, their sponsoring organizations and systems, and other health and related agencies and services operated as Catholic. It is an ecclesial community participating in the mission of the Catholic Church through its members' ministry of healing. CHA witnesses this ministry by providing leadership both within the Church and within the broader society and through its programs of education, facilitation, and advocacy.

John F. Tuohey, PhD, a priest of the Diocese of Springfield, MA, is a visiting assistant professor of moral theology, Department of Religion & Religious Education, School of Religious Studies, The Catholic University of America, Washington, DC. He received his doctorate in religious studies at the University of Louvain, Belgium.

Fr. Tuohey has published in such professional publications as *The American Journal of Hospice Care* and *The New Catholic Encyclopedia*. He has consulted in the areas of bioethics and moral theology, served as ethicist on the medical-moral committee at Mercy Hospital, Springfield, MA, and worked with the palliative care unit of Western Massachusetts Hospital and Hospice of Hampshire County.